# Updates in Anxiety Treatment

*Editors*

JEFFREY R. STRAWN
JUSTINE LARSON

# CHILD AND ADOLESCENT PSYCHIATRIC CLINICS OF NORTH AMERICA

www.childpsych.theclinics.com

*Consulting Editor*
JUSTINE LARSON

July 2023 • Volume 32 • Number 3

# ELSEVIER

1600 John F. Kennedy Boulevard • Suite 1800 • Philadelphia, Pennsylvania, 19103-2899

http://www.theclinics.com

**CHILD AND ADOLESCENT PSYCHIATRIC CLINICS OF NORTH AMERICA Volume 32, Number 3**
**July 2023 ISSN 1056–4993, ISBN-13: 978-0-443-18282-2**

Editor: Megan Ashdown
Developmental Editor: Arlene Campos

*Child and Adolescent Psychiatric Clinics of North America* (ISSN 1056-4993) is published quarterly by Elsevier Inc., 360 Park Avenue South, New York, NY 10010-1710. Months of issue are January, April, July, and October. Business and Editorial Offices: 1600 John F. Kennedy Boulevard, Suite 1800, Philadelphia, PA 19103-2899. Periodicals postage paid at New York, NY and additional mailing offices. Subscription prices are $369.00 per year (US individuals), $709.00 per year (US institutions), $100.00 per year (US & Canadian students), $411.00 per year (Canadian individuals), $862.00 per year (Canadian institutions), $473.00 per year (international individuals), $709.00 per year (international institutions), and $200.00 per year (international students). International air speed delivery is included in all *Clinics* subscription prices. All prices are subject to change without notice. **POSTMASTER:** Send address changes to *Child and Adolescent Psychiatric Clinics of North America*, Elsevier Health Sciences Division, Subscription Customer Service, 3251 Riverport Lane, Maryland Heights, MO 63043. **Customer Service: 1-800-654-2452 (U.S. and Canada); 314-447-8871 (outside U.S. and Canada). Fax: 314-447-8029. E-mail:** JournalsCustomer Service-usa@elsevier.com **(for print support) or** journalsonlinesupport-usa@elsevier.com **(for online support).**

*Reprints.* For copies of 100 or more of articles in this publication, please contact the Commercial Reprints Department, Elsevier Inc., 360 Park Avenue South, New York, New York 10010-1710 Tel.: 212-633-3874; Fax: 212-633-3820, E-mail: reprints@elsevier.com.

*Child and Adolescent Psychiatric Clinics of North America* is covered in *MEDLINE/PubMed (Index Medicus), ISI, SSCI, Research Alert, Social Search, Current Contents,* and *EMBASE/Excerpta Medica.*

# Contributors

## CONSULTING EDITOR

**JUSTINE LARSON, MD, MPH, DFAACAP**
Medical Director, Schools and Residential Treatment, Consulting Editor, *Child and Adolescent Psychiatric Clinics of North America*, Sheppard Pratt, Rockville, Maryland


## EDITORS

**JEFFREY R. STRAWN, MD**
Professor of Psychiatry, Pediatrics, and Clinical Pharmacology, Department of Psychiatry and Behavioral Neuroscience, Director, Anxiety Disorders Research Program, Co-Director, Center for Clinical and Translational Science and Training, University of Cincinnati College of Medicine, Divisions of Child and Adolescent Psychiatry and Clinical Pharmacology, Department of Pediatrics, Cincinnati Children's Hospital Medical Center, Cincinnati, Ohio

**JUSTINE LARSON, MD, MPH, DFAACAP**
Medical Director, Schools and Residential Treatment, Consulting Editor, *Child and Adolescent Psychiatric Clinics of North America*, Sheppard Pratt, Rockville, Maryland


## AUTHORS

**GREESHMA AGASTHYA, PhD**
Research Scientist, Computational Sciences and Engineering Division, Advanced Computing for Health Sciences Section, Oak Ridge National Laboratory, Oak Ridge, Tennessee

**CHERYL S. AL-MATEEN, MD, DFAPA, FAACAP**
Professor, Departments of Psychiatry and Pediatrics, Virginia Commonwealth University, Richmond, Virginia

**ROBERT T. AMMERMAN, PhD**
Professor, Division of Behavioral Medicine and Clinical Psychology, Department of Pediatrics, Cincinnati Children's Hospital Medical Center, Cincinnati, Ohio

**W. THOMAS BAUMEL, MD**
Department of Psychiatry and Behavioral Neuroscience, Anxiety Disorders Research Program, College of Medicine, University of Cincinnati, Cincinnati, Ohio

**JENNIFER B. BLOSSOM, PhD**
Assistant Professor, Department of Psychology, University of Maine, Orono, Maine

**ISABELLA C. BROWN, MA**
Doctoral Student, Berkeley School of Education, University of California, Berkeley, Berkeley, California

**MEGAN D. CHOCHOL, MD**
Assistant Professor, Department of Psychiatry, University of Utah and Huntsman Mental Health Institute, Salt Lake City, Utah

**MICHELE COSBY, PsyD. LCP**
Assistant Professor, Clinical Psychologist, Department of Psychiatry, Virginia Commonwealth University, Richmond, Virginia

**PAUL E. CROARKIN, DO, MS**
Professor of Psychiatry, Department of Psychiatry and Psychology, Mayo Clinic, Rochester, Minnesota

**ERIN DILLON-NAFTOLIN, MD**
Clinical Associate Professor, Partnership Access Line, Seattle Children's, Child and Adolescent Psychiatry and Behavioral Medicine, University of Washington, Child and Adolescent Psychiatry, Seattle, Washington

**LISA R. FORTUNA, MD, MPH**
Professor, Department of Psychiatry and Behavioral Sciences, University of California, San Francisco, Zuckerberg San Francisco General Hospital, San Francisco, California

**WILLIAM FRENCH, MD**
Associate Professor, Partnership Access Line, Seattle Children's, Child and Adolescent Psychiatry and Behavioral Medicine, University of Washington, Child and Adolescent Psychiatry, Seattle, Washington

**KRITI GANDHI, MD**
Assistant Professor, Department of Psychiatry, Children's National Hospital, Takoma Theatre, Washington, DC

**TRACY A. GLAUSER, MD**
Professor, Department of Pediatrics, Cincinnati Children's Hospital Medical Center, Cincinnati, Ohio

**ANDREW G. GUZICK, PhD**
Assistant Professor, Psychology, Psychiatry and Behavioral Sciences, Baylor College of Medicine, Houston, Texas

**JONATHAN HERSHFIELD, LCMFT**
Director, Center for OCD and Anxiety, Sheppard Pratt, Baltimore, Maryland

**JLYNN HOLLAND-CECIL, MS**
Fifth Year Clinical Health Psychology Doctoral Student, Virginia State University, Petersburg, Virginia

**NATHANIEL JUNGBLUTH, PhD**
Clinical Psychologist, Partnership Access Line, Seattle Children's, Seattle, Washington

**MICHAEL KEITER, BS**
Fourth Year Medical Student, Virginia Commonwealth University, Richmond, Virginia

**CRYSTAL LEWIS, BS**
Fourth Year Medical Student, Virginia Commonwealth University, Richmond, Virginia

**GESEAN G. LEWIS WOODS, MA**
Doctoral Student, Berkeley School of Education, University of California, Berkeley, Berkeley, California

**STELLA LOPEZ, PsyD, LCP**
Clinical Psychologist and Assistant Professor, Department of Psychiatry, Virginia Treatment Center for Children, VCU Health, Richmond, Virginia

**CASSANDRA M. NICOTRA, DO**
Child and Adolescent Psychiatry Fellow, Department of Pediatrics, Division of Child and Adolescent Psychiatry, Cincinnati Children's Hospital Medical Center, Cincinnati, Ohio

**JOHN P. PESTIAN, PhD**
Professor, Department of Pediatrics, Cincinnati Children's Hospital Medical Center, Cincinnati, Ohio

**MICHELLE V. PORCHE, EdD**
Associate Professor, Department of Psychiatry and Behavioral Sciences, University of California, San Francisco, San Francisco, California

**DIMAL D. SHAH, MD**
Assistant Clinical Professor, Department of Psychiatry, Virginia Commonwealth University, Richmond, Virginia

**MICHAEL SHAPIRO, MD, DFAPA, DFAACAP**
Associate Professor, Department of Psychiatry, University of Florida, Gainesville, Florida

**JORDAN T. STIEDE, MS**
Baylor College of Medicine, Houston, Texas

**ERIC A. STORCH, PhD**
McIngvale Presidential Endowed Chair & Professor Vice Chair & Head of Psychology Menninger Department of Psychiatry and Behavioral Sciences Baylor College of Medicine, Houston, Texas

**JEFFREY R. STRAWN, MD**
Professor of Psychiatry, Pediatrics, and Clinical Pharmacology, Department of Psychiatry and Behavioral Neuroscience, Director, Anxiety Disorders Research Program, Co-Director, Center for Clinical and Translational Science and Training, University of Cincinnati College of Medicine, Divisions of Child and Adolescent Psychiatry and Clinical Pharmacology, Department of Pediatrics, Cincinnati Children's Hospital Medical Center, Cincinnati, Ohio

**ERIKA S. TRENT, MA**
University of Houston, Houston, Texas

**ANDRES G. VIANA, PhD**
Associate Professor, Child Temperament Thoughts and Emotions Laboratory, Department of Psychology, University of Houston, Houston, Texas

**EMILY N. WARNER, MD, MPH**
Department of Psychiatry and Behavioral Neuroscience, University of Cincinnati College of Medicine, Cincinnati, Ohio

# Contents

This review summarizes risk factors for developing anxiety disorders in children and adolescents. A surfeit of risk factors, including temperament, family environment (eg, parenting style), environmental exposures (eg, particulate matter), and cognitive factors (eg, threat bias), increases the risk of anxiety in children. These risk factors can significantly impact the trajectory of pediatric anxiety disorders. The impact of severe acute respiratory syndrome COVID-19 2 infection on anxiety disorders in children is discussed in addition to its public health implications. Identifying risk factors for pediatric anxiety disorders creates a scaffold for the development of prevention strategies and for reducing anxiety-related disability.

This review summarizes the developmental epidemiology of childhood and adolescent anxiety disorders. It discusses the COVID-19 pandemic, sex differences, longitudinal course, and stability of anxiety disorders in addition to recurrence and remission. The trajectory of anxiety disorders— whether homotypic (ie, the same anxiety disorder persists over time) or heterotypic (ie, an anxiety disorder shifts to a different diagnosis over time) is discussed with regard to social, generalized, and separation anxiety disorders as well as specific phobia, and panic disorder. Finally, strategies for early recognition, prevention, and treatment of disorders are discussed.

The primary objective of this article is to consider the impact of the COVID-19 pandemic on pediatric anxiety from both a clinical and system-of-care lens. This includes illustrating the impact of the pandemic on pediatric anxiety disorders and consideration of factors important for special populations, including children with disabilities and learning differences. We consider the clinical, educational, and public health implications for addressing mental health needs like anxiety disorders and how we might promote better outcomes, particularly for vulnerable children and youth.

Anxiety disorders are the most common class of psychiatric conditions among children and adolescents. The cognitive behavioral model of childhood anxiety has a strong theoretic and empirical foundation that provides the basis for effective treatment. Cognitive behavioral therapy (CBT), with an emphasis on exposure therapy, is the gold standard treatment for childhood anxiety disorders, with strong empirical support. A case vignette demonstrating CBT for childhood anxiety disorders in practice, as well as recommendations for clinicians, are also provided.

Psychodynamic psychotherapy can be an effective treatment of pediatric anxiety disorders. Psychodynamic formulation can be easily integrated with other conceptualizations of anxiety (eg, biological/genetic, developmental, and social learning theory). Psychodynamic formulation helps determine whether anxiety symptoms represent innate biological responses, learned responses from early experiences, or defensive reactions to intrapsychic conflict. Child and Adolescent Anxiety Psychodynamic Psychotherapy and Psychoanalytic Child Therapy are two evidence-based manualized psychodynamic approaches to treating pediatric anxiety disorders.

The evidence base for psychopharmacologic interventions in children and adolescents with anxiety disorders has significantly increased, and our understanding of the relative efficacy and tolerability of interventions has expanded contemporaneously. Selective serotonin reuptake inhibitors (SSRIs) are the first-line pharmacologic treatment for pediatric anxiety due to their robust efficacy although other agents may have efficacy. This review summarizes the data concerning the use of SSRIs, serotonin and norepinephrine reuptake inhibitors (SNRIs), tricyclic antidepressants, atypical anxiolytics (eg, $5HT_{1A}$ agonists, alpha agonists), and benzodiazepines in pediatric anxiety disorder cases (ie, generalized anxiety disorder, separation anxiety disorder, social anxiety disorder, and panic disorder). The extant data suggest that SSRIs and SNRIs are effective and well tolerated. SSRIs as monotherapy and SSRIs + cognitive behavioral therapy reduce symptoms in youth with anxiety disorders. However, randomized controlled trials do not suggest efficacy for benzodiazepines or the $5HT_{1A}$ agonist, buspirone, in pediatric anxiety disorder cases.

Both pharmacologic and psychotherapeutic treatment-related changes increase activity in brain regions implicated in prefrontal regulatory circuits, and the functional connectivity of these regions with the amygdala is enhanced following pharmacological treatment. This may suggest overlapping mechanisms of action across therapeutic modalities. The existing literature is best viewed as a partially constructed scaffold on which to construct a vigorous understanding of biomarkers in pediatric anxiety syndromes. As the field approaches leveraging "fingerprints" in neuroimaging with "outputs" in neuropsychiatric tasks and scale, we can move beyond one-size-fits-all selection of psychiatric interventions toward more nuanced therapeutic strategies that recognize individual differences.

# CHILD AND ADOLESCENT PSYCHIATRIC CLINICS

---

**SERIES OF RELATED INTEREST**
Psychiatric Clinics
https://www.psych.theclinics.com/
Pediatric Clinics
https://www.pediatric.theclinics.com/

---

AACAP Members: Please go to www.jaacap.org for information on access to the Child and Adolescent Psychiatric Clinics. *Resident* Members of AACAP: Special access information is available at www.childpsych.theclinics.com.

---

**THE CLINICS ARE AVAILABLE ONLINE!**
Access your subscription at:
www.theclinics.com

# Preface

# Anxiety Disorders and Their Treatment in Youth: A New Era

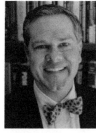 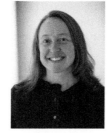

Jeffrey R. Strawn, MD     Justine Larson, MD, MPH
*Editors*

In the decade since pediatric anxiety disorders were last reviewed in the *Child and Adolescent Psychiatric Clinics of North America*, our field has seen tremendous advances. We re-classified the anxiety disorders in DSM-5, enhanced our understanding of the epidemiology neurobiology anxiety disorders. The evidence for both psychotherapeutic and psychopharmacologic treatment has been buttressed by dozens of additional trials. Beyond this, we have an evolving understanding of the morbidity of anxiety disorders and their role as substrates for the emergence of other disorders. Further, the COVID-19 pandemic increased the prevalence of pediatric anxiety disorders. Based on this increased recognition of the importance of anxiety disorders, their morbidity and increasing prevalence, in 2022, the US Prevention and Screening Task Force recommended that all youth between the ages of 8 and 18 years be screened for anxiety disorders. These events instantiate increased recognition of anxiety disorders and an appreciation of their keystone role within developmental psychopathology. Thus, this issue of the *Child and Adolescent Psychiatric Clinics of North America* is timely and immediately relevant to clinicians treating children and adolescents.

This issue begins with a review of the developmental context of anxiety in children and adolescents, including the distinct trajectories of anxiety disorders and the way in which they intercalate with developmentally appropriate, "normal" anxiety, with the latter characterized as proportional and expected. We also discuss how an increased understanding of the child and adolescent world, including his or her family environment, trauma, and biologic and environmental risk factors, interacts to produce resiliency or risk for developing anxiety disorders.

The stage having been set by a review of the developmental epidemiology and risk factors for anxiety disorders, the later works in this volume shift to a multidimensional understanding of anxiety disorders, including social and electronic media and racial

Child Adolesc Psychiatric Clin N Am 32 (2023) xi–xii
https://doi.org/10.1016/j.chc.2023.03.001
1056-4993/23/© 2023 Published by Elsevier Inc.

and cultural aspects of anxiety disorders. This is followed by several treatment-focused contributions on cognitive behavioral psychotherapy, psychodynamic psychotherapy, and pharmacotherapy for treating anxiety disorders in children and adolescents. However, these sections, which also include a contribution on the neurobiological effects of treatment in anxiety disorders, don't simply present the evidence that a particular treatment is effective. Rather, they focus on helping clinicians understand why and in whom a particular psychotherapeutic or psychopharmacologic intervention may be most helpful and how to tailor these interventions for individual patients. In essence, what sets these apart from many practice guidelines and reviews is that they provide a nuanced approach to the patient rather than a "one-size-fits-all" approach to diagnosing and treating anxiety disorders in children and adolescents.

Jeffrey R. Strawn, MD
Anxiety Disorders Research Program
Department of Psychiatry & Behavioral Neuroscience
University of Cincinnati, College of Medicine
260 Stetson Street, Suite 3200
Cincinnati, OH 45219, USA

Justine Larson, MD, MPH
Sheppard Pratt
4915 Aspen Hill Road
Rockville, MD 20853, USA

E-mail addresses:
strawnjr@uc.edu (J.R. Strawn)
Justine.Larson1@sheppardpratt.org (J. Larson)

# Risk Factors for Pediatric Anxiety Disorders

Emily N. Warner, MD, MPH[a],*, Jeffrey R. Strawn, MD[a,b]

## KEYWORDS

- Anxiety • Risk factors • Genetic biomarkers • Predispose • COVID-19 • Cognitive
- Internalizing

## KEY POINTS

- Risk factors for anxiety disorders in children and adolescents include cognitive, family environmental factors, sleep quality, substance use, genetic, and environmental toxicants.
- In youth, specific risk factors (eg, threat bias, externalizing disorders, genetic predispositions) interact to increase the risk of developing an anxiety disorder.
- Parental anxiety and personality, along with the family environment, may increase the risk of anxiety disorders in childhood.
- Several genetic risk factors have been identified for generalized anxiety disorder, specific phobia, social anxiety, and panic disorders.

## INTRODUCTION

A surfeit of risk factors, including genetics, temperament, cognition, and exposure to trauma, increase the risk of anxiety and anxiety disorders in children and adolescents. These risk factors include maladaptive responses to common situations and stressors as well as family environment (eg, parenting style), environmental exposures (eg, particulate matter), and cognitive factors (eg, threat bias). Understanding these risk factors and the way in which they interact is critical not only for primary and secondary prevention of anxiety disorders but also to increase knowledge regarding the maintenance of anxiety disorders, the persistence of residual symptoms, and their recurrence.

This article reviews risk factors for anxiety disorders in children and adolescents and highlights genetic biomarkers that predispose individuals to anxiety disorders.

[a] Department of Psychiatry and Behavioral Neuroscience, University of Cincinnati College of Medicine; Cincinnati, OH 45219, USA; [b] Divisions of Child & Adolescent Psychiatry and Clinical Pharmacology, Department of Pediatrics, Cincinnati Children's Hospital Medical Center, Cincinnati, OH, USA
* Corresponding author. Department of Psychiatry, Box 670559, 260 Stetson Street, Suite 3200, Cincinnati, OH 45267-0559.
E-mail address: warnerey@mail.uc.edu

Child Adolesc Psychiatric Clin N Am 32 (2023) 485–510
https://doi.org/10.1016/j.chc.2022.10.001
1056-4993/23/© 2022 Elsevier Inc. All rights reserved.
childpsych.theclinics.com

Identifying both the environmental and genetic basis of these disorders can have major implications on future prevention and treatment strategies.

## RISK FACTORS FOR THE DEVELOPMENT OF PEDIATRIC ANXIETY DISORDERS

A myriad of risk factors, including cognitive, environmental, genetic, and developmental causes have been identified in contributing to pediatric anxiety disorder development. Many of these risk factors can be identified in childhood and can predispose individuals to persistent anxiety later in life.

### Cognitive Risk Factors

From a cognitive perspective, bias toward threat-related stimuli, behavioral inhibition, intolerance of uncertainty, distress intolerance, and learned behaviors, such as avoidance and repetitive negative thinking, represent the most studied cognitive risk factors for developing anxiety disorders. These maladaptive cognitive responses to negative affect are associated with impaired emotion regulation and predict increased anxiety or a greater risk of developing anxiety disorders.

### Threat Bias

A hallmark of anxiety disorders is threat bias, an attentional bias toward threat-related stimuli. This exaggerated and selective attention to threat may underlie the development and maintenance of anxiety disorders. Children with anxiety disorders have a greater attentional bias toward threat-related stimuli compared with healthy controls, although this may be to a lesser degree than in adults.[1] A "moderation model" has been proposed in which all young children, including those between 5 months and 5 years, display biases toward threatening information.[2–4] As children develop, differences in attentional bias begin to develop. Children without anxiety inhibit an automatic threat response and respond in a cognitively controlled manner, whereas anxious children continue to display threat-related attentional bias. Thus, the difference in threat bias between children with anxiety and control children appears to increase with age. This trend was confirmed in a recent meta-analysis showing that children with anxiety may be less likely to develop effective top–down cognitive control in attentional and inhibitory processes as they mature. In other words, the attentional biases that are present in children at a young age continue to persist well into adolescence among anxious children.[1] This persistence of threat bias into adolescence and adulthood primes individuals for a hypervigilant response, even among common situations, and contributes to the development of anxiety disorders.

### Behavioral Inhibition

Behavioral inhibition—the tendency to withdraw from unfamiliar situations and experience distress in unknown environments—is highly heritable[5] and represents a significant risk factor for developing anxiety disorders. In toddlers, behavioral inhibition may manifest as agitation and distress to novel stimuli, whereas preschoolers have increased hesitancy and restraint in unfamiliar situations. However, behavioral inhibition is relatively stable. In other words, it does not change significantly from toddlerhood to early adulthood.[6,7] Behavioral inhibition strongly predicts the development of multiple anxiety disorders. It increases the risk of developing social anxiety disorder by seven-fold,[8] doubles the risk of developing generalized anxiety disorder and nearly doubles the risk of developing a specific phobia.[9]

   Early behavioral inhibition in childhood also predicts distinct associations between anxiety symptoms and attention-related amygdala-prefrontal cortex (PFC) circuitry across development.[10] Amygdala-PFC connectivity is associated with threat-related attention orienting, which is consistently implicated in neuroimaging studies of anxiety and anxiety disorders in youth.[11,12] There are two distinct developmental trajectories with regard to this. In the first, children with a history of high behavioral inhibition have anxiety symptoms that became more negatively correlated with DLPFC-amygdala connectivity as they aged when processing salient threats. In the second, the opposite pattern was observed. Children with a history of low behavioral inhibition have anxiety symptoms that became more positively correlated with DLPFC-amygdala activity over time.[10] This suggests that different childhood behavioral inhibition levels predict different trajectories of neurodevelopmental anxiety across the lifespan.

### Distress Intolerance

Distress intolerance, also referred to as affect or emotional intolerance, is characterized by a reduced ability to withstand uncomfortable situations and emotional states. Distress intolerance may maintain anxiety and internalizing disorders and has been linked to maladaptive emotion regulation strategies, such as avoidance. Greater youth-reported affect intolerance was strongly associated with youth-reported anxiety.[13] This supports previous research showing that low distress tolerance at baseline predicted greater perceived stress, which further increased youth-reported internalizing symptoms.[14] Distress intolerance represents a core process involved in developing and maintaining anxiety disorders in children and adolescents.

### Anxiety Sensitivity

Anxiety sensitivity involves the fear of sensations associated with the experience of anxiety and misinterpretation of these sensations as dangerous. For example, a child might fear the sensation of an increase in heart rate during an unfamiliar situation and interpret this as a sign of something more serious. In adults, anxiety sensitivity, like distress intolerance, increases the risk of internalizing symptoms, and specifically panic attacks.[15,16] Although there are fewer data in children, higher anxiety sensitivity is associated with greater anxiety in youth, including generalized, social and separation anxiety as well as panic. Anxiety sensitivity is also higher in youth with anxiety than those without an anxiety disorder.[17] In a different study, high anxiety sensitivity at age 11 predicted greater anxiety and depression in mid-to-late adolescence.[18] Distress intolerance and anxiety sensitivity represent components of affect intolerance vulnerability factor that increase the risk of developing anxiety disorders in youth.[13]

### Intolerance of Uncertainty

An inability to tolerate uncertainty involves a set of negative beliefs about uncertain situations. This leads to the avoidance of unfamiliar and uncertain situations and a tendency to react negatively to these circumstances on an emotional, cognitive, and behavioral level. At the core of intolerance of uncertainty is the fear of the unknown. Individuals with high intolerance of uncertainty are more prone to engage in worry and cognitive avoidance. Consistent with studies in adults,[19] greater intolerance of uncertainty predicts more anxiety in children and adolescents. Specifically, generalized anxiety disorder (GAD) is closely linked with the intolerance of uncertainty in children.[20,21] However, additional associations have been found between intolerance of uncertainty and social and separation anxiety disorders, panic disorder, obsessive-compulsive disorder, and health-related anxiety.[22-26] Despite evidence of association with GAD, several studies have found that intolerance of uncertainty contributed to overall worry among youth but not GAD severity.[27] These findings suggest that intolerance to uncertainty represents a transdiagnostic cognitive risk factor for anxiety and global anxiety severity.

### Repetitive Negative Thinking

Repetitive negative thinking has been linked to underlying worry regarding social interactions in children and adolescents. Numerous studies have shown that negative anticipatory processing and post-event processing have been found to predict social anxiety disorder,[24,28–31] GAD,[24] and high social phobia.[32,33] These findings were supported by Esbjorn and colleagues,[34] who found that a repetitive negative thinking pattern was a predictor of GAD. Children with frequent and severe repetitive negative thinking may not believe they can stop the cycle of worry and may therefore feel less in control of their thoughts. This leads to more uncertainty and negatively reinforces their anxiety. In addition, repetitive negative thinking is associated with more executive functioning problems in youth.[35] Overall, enhanced repetitive negative thinking in youth across several different anxiety disorders suggests a transdiagnostic role in this cognitive risk factor.[36]

### Executive Functioning

Executive functioning is defined as higher-order neurocognitive processes which underlie goal-directed behavior. In other words, it is a set of cognitive processes that include tasks such as top–down attention, error monitoring, information processing, working memory, and task switching. Evidence suggests that executive function is disrupted across multiple domains among anxious youth. This includes decreased cognitive flexibility and verbal working memory among children with anxiety disorders compared with nonanxious children.[37] Specifically, there are differences in functional activity within PFC regions such as the dorsolateral PFC,[38] anterior cingulate, frontal pole, and insula[39] as well as the organization and connectivity of the ventral attention, default mode,[40] and cingulo-opercular networks.[39] Compared with healthy adolescents, adolescents with GAD exhibit hyperactivity within the ventrolateral PFC and aberrant connections with other prefrontal regions during attentional tasks with emotional and neutral distractors.[41] In a heterogenous group of youths with an OCD or GAD, the dorsolateral PFC activity decreased during error processing compared with healthy youths.[38] Overall, executive function deficits among adolescents with GAD may impair cognitive capacity and negatively affect interpersonal functioning, which could exacerbate anxiety over time.[42,43] However, it is not well-established if deficits in executive function lead to anxiety disorders or if anxiety disorders themselves lead to executive functioning deficits. Additional research is needed to understand these associations better.

### Parental Disorders and the Risk of Developing Anxiety Disorders

Parental anxiety disorders increase the risk of offspring developing anxiety disorders. These disorders include internalizing disorders, such as GAD, social anxiety, and depression, as well as personality disorders.

### Parental Internalizing Disorders

Internalizing symptoms in both mothers and fathers are associated with increased childhood anxiety ratings.[44] Specifically, having a parent with an anxiety disorder has been associated with an increased risk of the development of anxiety disorders in offspring.[45] Parental GAD increases the risk of children developing GAD and other anxiety disorders.[46] The children of mothers with high levels of anxiety also show more difficulty tolerating distress.[47] Like parental anxiety, parental depression also increases the risk of pediatric anxiety disorders.[48] Specifically, associations between maternal depression and child internalizing behaviors emerge when maternal depression is chronic as opposed to time-limited.[49,50] Overall, when both parents experience increased depressive symptoms, children are more likely to develop anxiety and behavioral problems.[51] Given this association, clinicians may consider assessing parental internalizing symptoms and underlying disorders when evaluating and treating anxious children.[52]

### Parental Social Anxiety

Social anxiety disorder is highly heritable[53–55] and a child's risk of developing social anxiety disorder is nearly five times higher when they have a parent with social anxiety disorder.[53] Further, lifetime social anxiety disorder severity in parents is related to anxious behaviors and avoidance in children during their preschool years.[56] Poole and colleagues[57] examined the influence of familial vulnerability (eg, parent with social anxiety disorder) and child biological stress vulnerability (eg, cortisol reactivity to a social stressor) and found that children with heightened cortisol reactivity who had a parent with social anxiety disorder were at the greatest risk for developing social anxiety disorder. This study considers both parent-level factors and child-level biological vulnerabilities when considering the development of social anxiety among children.

### Parental Personality

Parental personality predicts the development of childhood anxiety disorders and specifically, parental Cluster A (paranoid, schizoid, and schizotypal personality) and C traits (avoidant, dependent and obsessive-compulsive personality) increased this risk. Interestingly, the impact of parental Cluster A traits on children is age-dependent, and may have the largest impact on school-aged children.[58] Parents with cluster A traits may attempt to influence or control their children more commonly than those without these traits, which may negatively impact children with increasing age and autonomy. Parents with Cluster C traits are also more likely to engage in more controlling parenting,[59] whereas those with Cluster B traits are more likely to be associated with childhood depression.

### Family Environment and the Risk of Developing Anxiety Disorders

### Overcontrolling environment

A family environment that is "overcontrolling" with parental overprotection may increase the risk of developing anxiety.[60–62] This parenting style conveys to the child that there is a constant threat, which can lead to hypervigilance and increased fear.[63] In addition, children exposed to this type of family environment may be less willing to explore their environment or cope in threatening situations, leading to increased anxiety in uncertain situations.[64] When parents model anxious and overcontrolling behavior, children are more reluctant to explore new situations and display more avoidance behaviors leading to higher rates of anxiety and subsequent anxiety disorders.

### Demandingness and warmth

Parental demandingness is associated with increased rates of anxiety disorders among children. Demandingness reflects how much control parents attempt to exert over their children. Demandingness is associated with specific parenting styles (eg, authoritarian, authoritative styles) in contrast to permissive parenting styles. In a study by Lo and colleagues,[65] when parental demandingness was high, deficits in executive functioning significantly predicted greater anxiety symptoms. In contrast, when parental demandingness was low, the association between executive functioning deficits and anxiety was weaker. Thus, low parental demandingness may protect children from developing anxiety disorders and parental warmth during adolescence is associated with less anxiety in adulthood.[62]

### Parenting style
Parenting styles have been categorized as authoritarian, authoritative, and permissive and there are direct interactions between child anxiety and the parent–child relationship.[66,67] An authoritarian parenting style is one in which the parent focuses on obedience, discipline, and control that places high demands on children. Authoritarian parenting practices are associated with increased internalizing symptoms in children[68] and children of authoritarian parents report more personal, social, and school maladjustment, and more depression and anxiety.[69] In addition, school-age children who perceive their parents as authoritarian have more anxiety-related symptoms than children who perceive their parents as more democratic.[70]

### Attachment style
Attachment type between parent and child is one of the most important family factors in a child's emotional security and development. Children who experience a trusting and secure parental bond are more likely to trust others, become independent, and overcome adversity. By contrast, children with insecure attachment have less social competence, fewer social skills, and more difficulty with peer interactions.[71,72] Bowlby[73] first observed that early parent–child attachment style predicted later psychopathology in children and linked insecure attachment style in childhood to the development of anxiety disorders in children over time.[74]

Ambivalent attachment (a subtype of insecure attachment) is characterized by inconsistent responses from caregivers and a child's preoccupation with a caregiver's emotional availability. Ambivalently attached children may have anxious and angry behaviors toward their caregivers and insecure-ambivalent attachment has a stronger association with the development of anxiety than other forms of insecure attachment.[73,75,76] A longitudinal study following infants to adolescence found that less insecure attachment predicted more social anxiety in adolescence.[77] Taken together, more than 50 years of research suggests that insecure attachment (specifically the ambivalent subtype), increases the risk of a child developing an anxiety disorder.

## Adversity and the Risk of Developing Anxiety Disorders

### Adverse childhood experiences
Adverse childhood experiences (ACEs) increase cognitive and attentional vulnerability, increasing the likelihood of developing anxiety symptoms later in life. The cumulative impact of ACEs has been associated with many different mental health problems, as well as a specific association with the development of anxiety.[78] One cross-sectional study using data from the 2016 to 2017 National Survey of Children's Health revealed that caregiver reports of ACEs among children were associated with a significantly higher likelihood of anxiety and depressive symptoms. Specifically, children exposed to four or more ACEs had greater anxiety than children exposed to fewer than four ACEs. There was a differential association between ACEs and anxiety and depression, where associations were overall stronger with depression for almost all ACE categories.[79] Further evidence among college-aged students shows that early adversity was associated with worsening mental health over a semester. Specifically, a student with two or more ACEs was approximately twice as likely to meet screening criteria for an anxiety or depressive disorder, despite not meeting the criteria for these disorders in the prior semester.[80] Consequently, the number

of ACEs a child experiences may directly impact the risk of developing anxiety symptoms later in life.

Different types of ACEs and early life stressors differentially influence the development of anxiety. Physical abuse is associated with the severity of anxiety disorders, whereas sexual and emotional abuse are associated with an increased risk of panic disorder and agoraphobia.[81] Sexual abuse is associated with greater anxiety disorder severity[82] and correlates with the highest risk of overall psychopathology severity.[83]

### Chronic stress

Experiencing consistently stressful events as a child has been linked to the development and maintenance of anxiety in children.[84,85] Historically, Chorpita and Barlow[84] proposed that persistent stress in early life, particularly involving uncontrollable events (eg, abuse, neglect, or impoverished environments) makes children more likely to interpret future situations as uncontrollable. Numerous studies reveal that children with anxiety disorders experienced more chronic and enduring adversity and negative life events earlier in their lives,[86–88] although the relationship between these exposures and specific anxiety disorders is generally difficult to disentangle, with the exception of separation anxiety disorder. Children aged 7 to 12 years with separation anxiety disorder had more negative life events over the preceding 12 months compared with children with other anxiety disorders. These youth with separation anxiety disorder are also more likely to live with a single parent or experience frequent parental arguments, leading to more chronic stress.[89] Taken together, these findings suggest that chronic stress may influence the development of global anxiety burden and specifically increase the risk of developing separation anxiety disorder.

### Socioeconomic status

Poverty is associated with chronic stress and trauma, particularly among children. Previous studies have shown that children from lower socioeconomic status (SES) backgrounds are at higher risk of developing anxiety disorders.[90] In addition, individuals with from lower SES environments experience more anxiety symptoms after traumatic events compared with individuals from higher SES backgrounds.[91] In children living in poverty, more peripheral inflammation enhances threat-related amygdala activation and reward-related striatal activation.[92] This association may be due to chronic adversity experienced in low-income environments and links poverty to increased stress reactivity. These effects were more clearly seen during the recent COVID-19 pandemic, which affected the mental health of whole populations, but disproportionately affected those marginalized and in low-income communities. Therefore, an awareness of SES when treating anxious children is important, particularly given disparate mental health outcomes that have been further illustrated during the COVID-19 pandemic.

### Bullying

With 36% of youth reporting having been bullied,[93] we now recognize not only its prevalence but increasingly, the long-term sequelae of bullying. In a recent meta-analysis, being either a victim or perpetrator of bullying were strongly associated with later anxiety symptoms.[94] In addition, youth who were bullied between ages 7 to 11 were more likely to report anxiety (and depression) in early adulthood (age 23).[95] Further, cyberbullying victimization is associated with greater anxiety and depression.[96] Overall, different forms of bullying, both victimization, and perpetration, significantly increase the likelihood of developing anxiety.

### Externalizing disorders and the risk of developing anxiety disorders

Externalizing disorders—those conditions involving excessive overt and disruptive behaviors are generally categorized into "early" externalizing disorders with pre-pubertal onset (eg, oppositional defiant disorder [ODD], and attention-deficit hyperactivity disorder [ADHD]) and "late" externalizing disorders that emerge during or after adolescence (eg, conduct disorder, substance use disorders).[97] There is notable co-occurrence of externalizing disorders and anxiety disorders, with 30% to 60% of children with an early externalizing disorder also reporting an anxiety disorder, and vice versa (children with anxiety disorders reporting co-occurring externalizing disorder).[98] Clinically, "symptoms" of anxiety disorders could be related to the underlying anxiety disorder. For example, consider a child with separation and GADs who present irritability and frequent episodes of anger who argues with adults and "refuses to comply with request from authority figures." Irritability may relate to the underlying GAD and the episodes of anger or arguing if they occur during times of threatened separation (eg, bedtime, leaving for school) and would be better accounted for by the separation and GADs rather than ODD.

Early externalizing disorders may precede—and potentially increase the risk for developing—anxiety disorders.[99] Knappe and colleagues[100] followed 1053 adolescents (14–17 years) and assessed early and late externalizing disorders and anxiety disorders at baseline, two, four, and 10-year follow-ups. Adolescents with early externalizing disorders were at increased risk for later anxiety disorders (except for specific phobia preceding ADHD and GAD preceding conduct disorder) compared with children and adolescents without prior externalizing conditions.

Conversely, anxiety disorders more often preceded the onset of late externalizing disorders, partly due to increased risk-taking and overtly disruptive behaviors from childhood to adolescence. Thus, identifying early externalizing conditions, such as ODD, conduct disorder, and ADHD, and providing early treatment may help to mitigate the risk of anxiety disorder development.

### Attention-deficit hyperactivity disorder

Among externalizing disorders, ADHD is a significant risk factor for developing anxiety. The heterotypic continuity of anxiety and depressive symptoms may relate to underlying comorbidity with ADHD, ODD, and conduct disorder.[101] Further, early ADHD symptoms predict more anxiety disorder symptoms later in life, although this may also relate to overlapping anxiety and attentional symptoms.[102] As such, impaired executive functioning, particularly shifting attention and difficulty focusing, are present in ADHD and anxiety and may explain—in part—the association between the two disorders.[103] The association between ADHD and anxiety disorders may also relate to time-varying confounding variables; difficulties with peers or social exclusion in patients with ADHD may contribute to the development of anxiety symptoms.[104,105] Given this association, treating underlying ADHD early may decrease the risk of developing anxiety.

### Sleep disturbances and the risk of developing anxiety disorders

Sleep disturbances, across studies, predict later anxiety disorders.[106,107] In a longitudinal study of nearly 10,000 young women, sleep disturbances nearly tripled the risk of developing an anxiety disorder in early adulthood.[106] However, the relationship between sleep and anxiety may be bidirectional.[108,109] Neurobiologically, sleep deprivation—even for one night—increases amygdala activity and reduces its functional connectivity with the medial PFC. This reduced brain activation and functional connectivity diminish the ability to regulate anxiety following disrupted sleep.[110] Further, individuals with high trait anxiety experience moderate sleep problems, suggesting that anxiety contributes to disrupted sleep.[111] Bidirectional links were found between dysregulated sleep and internalizing symptoms in the follow-up study of children and adolescents with generalized, separation, and social anxiety disorders in the Child/Adolescent Anxiety Multimodal Extended Long-Term Study (CAMELS).[112] Further, poor sleep quality and duration predicted greater anxiety, depression, and externalizing symptoms among youth ages 8 to 13 over a 5-year follow-up, with less evidence for the relationship in the opposite direction.[113] Taken together, these findings underscore the need to address sleep-related difficulties, given that early poor sleep quality may predispose to increased anxiety later in life with the later potential for poor sleep and more severe anxiety to reverberate with one another.

### Substance use

Substance use, including alcohol and cannabis, is associated with an increased risk of developing anxiety disorders among adolescents. Specifically, greater alcohol use is associated with an increased risk of panic symptoms in adolescents and young adults.[114,115] This link between panic symptoms and alcohol use may relate to attempts by adolescents to use a central nervous system depressant (alcohol) as an anxiolytic—the self-medication hypothesis.[116] However, consuming alcohol is not always associated with a history of panic attacks suggesting that the self-medication hypothesis may not solely explain the relationship between alcohol use and panic symptoms or panic attacks. In addition, the physiologic arousal that occurs with repeated or heavy alcohol consumption combined with disruptions in neurologic function[117] may increase the risk for panic-related symptoms.[118] Interestingly, epigenetic studies have linked histone acetylation, methylation changes, and anxiety-like behavior following alcohol binges during adolescence[119] and administration of histone deacetylase inhibitors decreased anxiety-like behavior and ethanol consumption after adolescent ethanol exposure.[119,120] However, multicollinearity may also contribute to the relationship between alcohol use and panic symptoms during adolescents: experimentation with alcohol and other substances increases during adolescence, and symptoms of panic disorder typically emerge during this period.[121] For these reasons, it is important to assess the potential bidirectional association between alcohol use and the risk of panic disorder, particularly during adolescence.

Cannabis use, particularly daily use, in adolescence may increase the risk of developing anxiety disorders, even when individuals stop using cannabis. This suggests that early cannabis exposure creates a vulnerability to developing anxiety symptoms later in life, even among regular users who achieve abstinence.[122] Notably, during the COVID-19 pandemic, rates of adolescent alcohol and cannabis use increased, with approximately 50% engaging in substance use alone.[123,124] Interestingly, a lack of positive coping skills and potential neurobiological pathways may contribute to the relationship between stress, anxiety, and craving for substance use.[125] Therefore, increased substance use in adolescents could contribute to higher prevalence rates of anxiety disorders, particularly as we understand the post-COVID-19 pandemic sequelae.

### Environmental exposures

Less is known regarding environmental exposures that contribute to the development of pediatric anxiety disorders, such as air pollution.[126] However, according to a study by Brunst and colleagues,[127] traffic pollution was associated with increased generalized anxiety symptoms. Specifically, myo-inositol concentrations in the anterior cingulate cortex mediate the association between traffic-related air pollution and anxiety. More recently, specific components of air pollution that can induce oxidative stress and inflammation, such as particulate matter, have been linked to worsening anxiety disorders. Exposure to particulate matter with an aerodynamic diameter of <2.5 μm ($PM_{2.5}$) is associated with an increased risk of psychiatric emergency department visits for children and adolescents.[126] In addition, exposure to mercury and other toxicants is associated with an increased risk of developing anxiety disorders, even when correcting for maternal age, ethnicity, fish intake, household income, maternal education, and marital status. Evidence shows that cord and maternal blood mercury concentrations at birth are associated with more anxiety disorders at age 8 (when many anxiety disorders begin to emerge).[128] Thus, environmental exposures may play a vital role in neurodevelopment and behavioral outcomes among children. Assessing a child's physical environment is important when evaluating anxiety disorder risk.

### Coronavirus Disease-2019

### Psychosocial Stress

The COVID-19 pandemic created a worldwide mental health crisis. The pandemic's mental health toll is particularly significant in children and adolescents, as younger individuals may lack the same resilience and coping mechanisms as adults.[129] The prevalence of child and adolescent anxiety during the pandemic nearly doubled compared with pre-pandemic estimates, with rates of depression and anxiety around 25% and 20%, respectively.[130] The combination of loss of peer interactions, social isolation, and reduced contact with social support networks likely contributes to increasing anxiety in youth.[130,131] Overall, adolescents who perceived low rates of social support during the pandemic experienced more anxiety.[131] Further, from a psychosocial support standpoint, school-based psychological services—which serve many youth with anxiety and other psychiatric disorders—were unavailable when schools converted to virtual instruction.[132] This combination of social isolation and lack of support networks increased anxiety among youth during the COVID-19 pandemic.

### Association of Severe Acute Respiratory Syndrome Coronavirus 2, COVID-19, and Inflammation

Infections early in life increase the risk of developing several anxiety disorders, including panic disorder, social anxiety disorder, and GAD.[133] This risk relationship relates to myriad factors, including increased proinflammatory cytokines. Coronaviruses produce psychiatric symptoms through direct viral infection of the Central Nervous System or indirectly through an immune response.[134] Further, these viruses are neurotropic and can induce a "cytokine storm," leading to neuroinflammation and subsequent psychiatric symptoms.[135,136] In patients with acute COVID-19, interleukin (IL)-1β concentrations are higher in those with anxiety and depressive symptoms compared to those without.[137] In addition, in patients with severe acute respiratory syndrome coronavirus 2 (SARS-CoV-2) infection, the systemic-immune inflammation indices, based on peripheral platelet, neutrophil, and lymphocyte counts, were associated with increased anxiety at follow-up.[138] The relationship between SARS-CoV-2 infection or COVID-19 and anxiety symptoms or the development of an anxiety disorder is likely multifactorial; however, several studies suggest that an exaggerated inflammatory response may play a role in the development of anxiety.

## Genetic Risk Factors

The heritability of anxiety disorders varies based on the type of disorder, the complex inheritance, and many genetic variants that interact with other risk factors. Previously, candidate genes were the focus of molecular genetic research, particularly genes involved in monoaminergic transmission. However, a more recent meta-analysis showed only an association of panic disorder with *TMEM132D* gene variants and *NPSR1, HTR2A,* and *MAOA* genes.[139] Research has shifted toward genome-wide association studies with increased advances in low-cost genotyping. Some preliminary studies have shown only a few significant genome-wide loci. For example, a survey by Levey and colleagues examined anxiety in two million people and identified five significant genome-wide loci.[140] Even fewer studies have examined copy-number variants, with some data suggesting that some copy-number variants increase the risk of developing anxiety disorders.[141]

No single converging pathway has been identified from these initial genome-wide studies, and further research is required to investigate genetic risk factors for mental disorders. These new biological and genetic insights have significant implications for further understanding the onset and development of anxiety disorders and creating new treatments.

## Genetic Risk Factors for Generalized Anxiety Disorder

It is estimated that the heritability of GAD is roughly 35%.[142] Only a few studies have been conducted among patients with GAD to determine vulnerability genes for this population.[143] Previously, genes for monoamine oxidase A (*MAOA*) and solute carrier family six member 4 (*SLC6A4*) were identified as being potentially associated with the pathogenesis of GAD.[144,145] GAD has also been associated with a 5-hydroxytryptamine receptor 1A (*5-HTR1A*) gene variation, which has proven to be partially mediated by comorbidity with depression.[146]

A recent study[147] showed that the *Met* allele of the functional brain-derived neurotrophic factor (BDNF) *Val66Met* polymorphism, along with an increase in serum BDNF concentrations, increases the risk of developing GAD. However, the *Val66Met* association was not seen in individuals with GAD who were Han Chinese,[148] raising the possibility of ethnicity-related differences. Microarray studies of peripheral gene expression signatures have become a promising approach to identifying genetic risk factors and leveraging transcriptional and microRNA (miRNA) analysis. One specific miRNA array study using peripheral blood mononuclear cells (PBMCs) showed that levels of circulating miR-4505, miR-4484, miR-4674, miR-5103p, and miR-663 were upregulated in patients with GAD. However, the exact mechanism of this association requires further explanation.

In a different study by Wingo and colleagues,[149] generalized anxiety symptoms were associated with gene expression profiles (N = 336) and differed between anxious males and healthy controls, with 631 genes differentially expressed. Gene set enrichment analysis revealed that genes with altered expression levels in anxious males were involved in the response of various immune cells (monocytes, B-cells, and myeloid dendritic cells) to vaccination and acute infection. This suggests inflammatory pathways may predispose to the negative effects of GAD on physical health.

## Genetic Risk Factors for Panic Disorder

Linkage studies[150] suggest that chromosomal regions 13q, 14q, 22q, 4q31-q34, and 9q31 are associated with panic disorder. However, only a few genes have been

**Table 1**
Selected Risk Factors for Anxiety Disorders in Youth

| Risk Factor | Category | Description |
|---|---|---|
| Cognitive | Threat bias | • Attentional bias toward threat-related stimuli<br>• Anxious children show difficulty with top-down cognitive control |
| | Behavioral inhibition (BI) | • Withdraw from unfamiliar situations and experience distress<br>• Strongest association with social anxiety disorder<br>• Associated with increased risk of GAD and specific phobia<br>• Different childhood BI predict different trajectories of neurodevelopmental anxiety |
| | Distress intolerance | • Reduced ability to withstand emotional distress<br>• Maladaptive emotion regulation (eg, avoidance)<br>• Low distress intolerance predicts greater stress |
| | Anxiety sensitivity | • Fear of sensations and misinterpretation of sensations as dangerous<br>• Increases risk of panic symptoms, GAD, social anxiety, and separation anxiety |
| | Intolerance of uncertainty | • Negative beliefs about uncertain situations<br>• Avoidance and fear of the unknown<br>• Positive association between intolerance of uncertainty and anxiety<br>• Increased risk of GAD, social anxiety, separation anxiety, panic disorder, OCD |
| | Repetitive negative thinking | • Predicts social anxiety disorder, GAD, and social phobia<br>• Unable to stop cycle of worry<br>• Increased uncertainty and lack of control |
| | Executive functioning | • Executive function disrupted among anxious youth<br>• Differences in functional activity within prefrontal regions |
| Parental disorders | Internalizing disorders<br>Social anxiety<br>Personality disorder | • Maternal/paternal anxiety and depression<br>• Social anxiety in parents predicts development in offspring<br>• Parents with Cluster A and C traits increase anxiety risk in youth |

|  |  |  |
|---|---|---|
| Family environment | Overcontrolling | • Parental overprotection<br>• Constant threat leading to hypervigilance and fear<br>• Less coping strategies and willingness to explore unknown |
| | Demandingness/warmth | • High demandingness led to deficits in executive functioning with increased anxiety risk<br>• Warmth is protective factor<br>• Authoritarian style predicts childhood anxiety |
| | Style<br>Attachment | • Insecure ambivalent attachment |
| Adversity | Adverse childhood experiences (ACE) | • Number of ACEs experienced in childhood may impact risk of anxiety development<br>• Physical, sexual, and emotional abuse are associated with different anxiety subtypes |
| | Chronic stress | • Uncontrollable events, abuse, neglect, impoverished environments<br>• Association with separation anxiety<br>• Poverty associated with increased chronic stress and trauma |
| | Socioeconomic status | • Specific inflammatory markers correlated with amygdala activation<br>• COVID-19 and additional stress |
| | Bullying | • Both victim and perpetrator<br>• Traditional and cyberbullying |
| Externalizing disorders | ADHD | • "Early" externalizing disorders (ODD, conduct, ADHD) predict anxiety development<br>• ADHD most significant externalizing disorder associated with anxiety risk |
| Sleep | | • Alcohol and cannabis use linked to increased anxiety<br>• Relationship between alcohol and panic disorder<br>• Increased rates of substance use among adolescents during COVID-19 |
| Substance | | • Alcohol and cannabis use linked to increased anxiety<br>• Relationship between alcohol and panic disorder<br>• Increased rates of substance use among adolescents during COVID-19 |
| Environmental | | • Traffic pollution<br>• Air pollution and particulate matter<br>• Mercury exposure<br>• Cord and maternal blood mercury concentrations at birth |

(continued on next page)

**Table 1**
*(continued)*

| Risk Factor | Category | Description |
|---|---|---|
| COVID-19 | Psychosocial inflammation | • Lack of positive coping skills<br>• Loss of peer interactions, increased social isolation, reduced social support networks (ie, school closures)<br>• Pro-inflammatory cytokines after COVID-19 infection<br>• Elevated (IL)-1β concentrations<br>• Systemic Immune Inflammation Index (SII) associated with increased anxiety rates |
| Genetic | | • Gene variants: *TMEM132D, NPSR1, HTR2A,* and *MAOA* genes<br>• Genome-wide association studies |
| | Generalized anxiety disorder (GAD) | • *MAOA* and *SLC6A4* genes<br>• *5-HTR1A* gene variation<br>• BDNF Val66Met polymorphism<br>• miRNA analysis |
| | Panic disorder | • chromosomal regions 13q, 14q, 22q, 4q31-q34, and 9q31<br>• Val158Met polymorphism of the COMT gene<br>• *TMEM132D* |
| | Specific phobia | • Epigenetic studies involving *MAOA, CRHR1,* and *OXTR*<br>• *MAOA* uVNTR alleles<br>• BDNF gene variant<br>• Familial vulnerability based on subtypes |
| | Social anxiety disorder | • Chromosome 16<br>• *SLCA2*<br>• *RGS2* SNPs predicted treatment patterns |

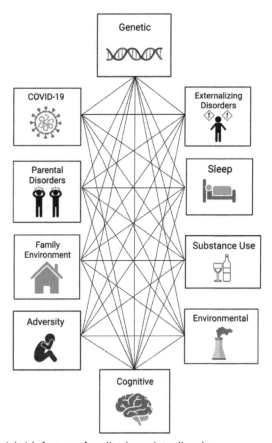

**Fig. 1.** Multifactorial risk factors of pediatric anxiety disorders.

associated with the risk of developing panic disorder within these loci. Specifically, the *Val158Met* polymorphism of the *COMT* gene increases panic disorder susceptibility in several studies, and this effect has been shown in a meta-analysis.[150] Importantly, association studies primarily focused on the "classic" candidate genes, such as genes related to serotonin, dopamine, or adenosine systems.[151] More recently, though, genes implicated in neuroendocrine, opioidergic, immune, and neurotrophic factors have been examined; however, results from candidate-gene association studies are inconsistent.

Howe and colleagues[139] conducted a meta-analysis of previous genetic association studies of panic disorder and examined 23 variants from 20 genes previously implicated in the susceptibility to panic disorder. Only two genes, *COMT* and *TMEM132D*, survived significant correction for multiple testing. In addition, hypothesis-driven studies, including investigations of epigenetic mechanisms (eg, differential methylation of genes), implicate *MAOA*,[152] *CRHR1*,[153] and *OXTR*[154] in the risk of developing panic disorder and social anxiety disorder. That these genes relate to monoaminergic function (*MAOA*), regulation of the hypothalamic-pituitary-adrenal axis (*CRHR1*), and the prosocial peptide oxytocin (*OXTR1*) is of interest and raises the possibility that early changes within these systems might play a key role in the development of anxiety disorders.

### Genetic Risk Factors for Specific Phobia

The risk of developing specific phobia has been associated with functional polymorphisms in the *MAO-A uVNTR* promoter gene. A trend for a more frequent presence of >3 repeat alleles of the *MAO-A* gene polymorphism among female patients with specific phobia was seen, suggesting a more active form of the MAO-A enzyme. This supports a possible role for MAO-A inhibitor action in anxiety disorders among females.[155] In addition, in Han Chinese patients with specific phobia, risk has been associated with BDNF gene variants.[156] Finally, meta-analyses of specific phobia risk suggest moderate heritability, although the heritability range varies across specific phobia subtypes.[157]

### Genetic Risk Factors for Social Anxiety Disorder

Gelernter and colleagues[158] found a significant linkage for SAD on chromosome 16. It was further hypothesized that as the gene encoding norepinephrine transporter *SLC6A2* maps to this broad region, this gene may influence the development of social anxiety disorder.

### SUMMARY

The risk for developing anxiety disorders in children and adolescents is multifactorial (**Table 1**). Specific risk factors include genetic, environmental, cognitive, and psychosocial risk factors, all of which interact (**Fig. 1**). In addition, certain risk factors may lead to specific anxiety disorders or participate in distinct risk trajectories. Recognizing these risk factors early or addressing these risk factors before anxiety disorders develop could represent primary prevention or secondary prevention strategy that could forestall the morbidity and mortality associated with anxiety disorders in youth. In addition, the COVID-19 pandemic and infection with SARS-CoV-2 represent the newest risk factor to be identified.

### CLINICS CARE POINTS

- Clinicians should carefully obtain family histories of anxiety disorders, particularly in the primary care setting, which could alert clinicians to patients at higher risk for developing anxiety.
- Addressing adversity, including adverse childhood experiences, chronic stress, and bullying is clinically important.
- Optimally treating certain externalizing disorders in children may mitigate the risk of subsequently developing anxiety disorders.
- Sleep and anxiety mutually influence one another.
- Increased substance use has been observed among adolescents during the COVID-19 pandemic, along with increased rates of anxiety.
- COVID-19 contributes to increased psychosocial stress, and severe acute respiratory syndrome coronavirus2 infection may worsen anxiety or contribute to the development of anxiety disorders.

### DISCLOSURE

Dr J R. Strawn has received research support from the Yung Family Foundation, the National Institutes of Health (NIMH/NIEHS), the National Center for Advancing

Translational Sciences, United States, the Patient Centered Outcomes Research Institute (PCORI), United States and Abbvie. He has received material support from Myriad Health and royalties from three texts (Springer) and has received honoraria from Neuroscience Education Institute, the American Academy of Child & Adolescent Psychiatry and the American Academy of Pediatric. Dr J R. Strawn serves as an author for *UpToDate* and an Associate Editor for *Current Psychiatry* and has provided consultation to the FDA, Cereval and IntraCellular Therapeutics. Views expressed within this article represent those of the authors and are not intended to represent the position of NIMH, the National Institutes of Health (NIH), United States, or the Department of Health and Human Services.

## ACKNOWLEDGMENTS

This work was supported by the Yung Family Foundation, the National Institutes of Health (NICHD, R01HD098757, R01HD099775, JRS).

## REFERENCES

1. Dudeney J, Sharpe L, Hunt C. Attentional bias towards threatening stimuli in children with anxiety: a meta-analysis. Clin Psychol Rev 2015;40:66–75.
2. Field AP, Lester KJ. Is there room for 'development' in developmental models of information processing biases to threat in children and adolescents? Clin Child Fam Psychol Rev 2010;13(4):315–32.
3. LoBue V. More than just another face in the crowd: superior detection of threatening facial expressions in children and adults. Dev Sci 2009;12(2):305–13.
4. Lobue V, DeLoache JS. Detecting the snake in the grass: attention to fear-relevant stimuli by adults and young children. Psychol Sci 2008;19(3):284–9.
5. Emde RN, Plomin R, Robinson JA, et al. Temperament, emotion, and cognition at fourteen months: the MacArthur Longitudinal Twin Study. Child Dev 1992; 63(6):1437–55.
6. Fox NA, Henderson HA, Marshall PJ, et al. Behavioral inhibition: linking biology and behavior within a developmental framework. Annu Rev Psychol 2005;56: 235–62.
7. Goldsmith HH, Lemery KS. Linking temperamental fearfulness and anxiety symptoms: a behavior-genetic perspective. Biol Psychiatry 2000;48(12): 1199–209.
8. Clauss JA, Blackford JU. Behavioral inhibition and risk for developing social anxiety disorder: a meta-analytic study. J Am Acad Child Adolesc Psychiatry 2012;51(10):1066–1075 e1.
9. Sandstrom A, Uher R, Pavlova B. Prospective association between childhood behavioral inhibition and anxiety: a meta-analysis. J Abnorm Child Psychol 2020;48(1):57–66.
10. Abend R, Swetlitz C, White LK, et al. Levels of early-childhood behavioral inhibition predict distinct neurodevelopmental pathways to pediatric anxiety. Psychol Med 2020;50(1):96–106.
11. Price RB, Allen KB, Silk JS, et al. Vigilance in the laboratory predicts avoidance in the real world: a dimensional analysis of neural, behavioral, and ecological momentary data in anxious youth. Dev Cogn Neurosci 2016;19:128–36.
12. White LK, Sequeira S, Britton JC, et al. Complementary features of attention bias modification therapy and cognitive-behavioral therapy in pediatric anxiety disorders. Am J Psychiatry 2017;174(8):775–84.

13. Shaw AM, Halliday ER, Tonarely NA, et al. Relationship of affect intolerance with anxiety, depressive, and obsessive-compulsive symptoms in youth. J Affect Disord 2021;280(Pt A):34–44.

14. Felton JW, Banducci AN, Shadur JM, et al. The developmental trajectory of perceived stress mediates the relations between distress tolerance and internalizing symptoms among youth. Dev Psychopathol 2017;29(4):1391–401.

15. Schmidt NB, Lerew DR, Jackson RJ. The role of anxiety sensitivity in the pathogenesis of panic: prospective evaluation of spontaneous panic attacks during acute stress. J Abnorm Psychol 1997;106(3):355–64.

16. Schmidt NB, Zvolensky MJ, Maner JK. Anxiety sensitivity: prospective prediction of panic attacks and Axis I pathology. J Psychiatr Res 2006;40(8):691–9.

17. Noel VA, Francis SE. A meta-analytic review of the role of child anxiety sensitivity in child anxiety. J Abnorm Child Psychol 2011;39(5):721–33.

18. Allan NP, Felton JW, Lejuez CW, et al. Longitudinal investigation of anxiety sensitivity growth trajectories and relations with anxiety and depression symptoms in adolescence. Dev Psychopathol 2016;28(2):459–69.

19. Osmanagaoglu N, Creswell C, Dodd HF. Intolerance of Uncertainty, anxiety, and worry in children and adolescents: a meta-analysis. J Affect Disord 2018;225: 80–90.

20. Read KL, Comer JS, Kendall PC. The Intolerance of Uncertainty Scale for Children (IUSC): discriminating principal anxiety diagnoses and severity. Psychol Assess 2013;25(3):722–9.

21. Donovan CL, Holmes MC, Farrell LJ. Investigation of the cognitive variables associated with worry in children with Generalised Anxiety Disorder and their parents. J Affect Disord 2016;192:1–7.

22. Boelen PA, Vrinssen I, van Tulder F. Intolerance of uncertainty in adolescents: correlations with worry, social anxiety, and depression. J Nerv Ment Dis 2010; 198(3):194–200.

23. Cornacchio D, Sanchez AL, Coxe S, et al. Factor structure of the intolerance of uncertainty scale for children. J Anxiety Disord 2018;53:100–7.

24. Hearn CS, Donovan CL, Spence SH, et al. Do worry and its associated cognitive variables alter following CBT treatment in a youth population with Social Anxiety Disorder? Results from a randomized controlled trial. J Anxiety Disord 2018;53: 46–57.

25. Hearn CS, Donovan CL, Spence SH, et al. What's the worry with social anxiety? Comparing cognitive processes in children with generalized anxiety disorder and social anxiety disorder. Child Psychiatry Hum Dev 2017;48(5):786–95.

26. Wright KD, Lebell MA, Carleton RN. Intolerance of uncertainty, anxiety sensitivity, health anxiety, and anxiety disorder symptoms in youth. J Anxiety Disord 2016;41:35–42.

27. Cowie J, Clementi MA, Alfano CA. Examination of the intolerance of uncertainty construct in youth with generalized anxiety disorder. J Clin Child Adolesc Psychol 2018;47(6):1014–22.

28. Asbrand J, Svaldi J, Kramer M, et al. Familial accumulation of social anxiety symptoms and maladaptive emotion regulation. PLoS One 2016;11(4): e0153153.

29. Keil V, Asbrand J, Tuschen-Caffier B, et al. Children with social anxiety and other anxiety disorders show similar deficits in habitual emotional regulation: evidence for a transdiagnostic phenomenon. Eur Child Adolesc Psychiatry 2017;26(7): 749–57.

30. Legerstee JS, Garnefski N, Jellesma FC, et al. Cognitive coping and childhood anxiety disorders. Eur Child Adolesc Psychiatry 2010;19(2):143–50.

31. Schmitz J, Kramer M, Blechert J, et al. Post-event processing in children with social phobia. J Abnorm Child Psychol 2010;38(7):911–9.

32. Klemanski DH, Curtiss J, McLaughlin KA, et al. Emotion regulation and the transdiagnostic role of repetitive negative thinking in adolescents with social anxiety and depression. Cognit Ther Res 2017;41(2):206–19.

33. Schmitz J, Kramer M, Tuschen-Caffier B. Negative post-event processing and decreased self-appraisals of performance following social stress in childhood social anxiety: an experimental study. Behav Res Ther 2011;49(11):789–95.

34. Esbjorn BH, Falch A, Walczak MA, et al. Social anxiety disorder in children: investigating the relative contribution of automatic thoughts, repetitive negative thinking and metacognitions. Behav Cogn Psychother 2021;49(2):159–71.

35. Mennies RJ, Stewart LC, Olino TM. The relationship between executive functioning and repetitive negative thinking in youth: a systematic review of the literature. Clin Psychol Rev 2021;88:102050.

36. Golombek K, Lidle L, Tuschen-Caffier B, et al. The role of emotion regulation in socially anxious children and adolescents: a systematic review. Eur Child Adolesc Psychiatry 2020;29(11):1479–501.

37. Toren P, Sadeh M, Wolmer L, et al. Neurocognitive correlates of anxiety disorders in children: a preliminary report. J Anxiety Disord 2000;14(3):239–47.

38. Fitzgerald KD, Liu Y, Stern ER, et al. Reduced error-related activation of dorsolateral prefrontal cortex across pediatric anxiety disorders. J Am Acad Child Adolesc Psychiatry 2013;52(11):1183–1191 e1.

39. Shanmugan S, Wolf DH, Calkins ME, et al. Common and dissociable mechanisms of executive system dysfunction across psychiatric disorders in youth. Am J Psychiatry 2016;173(5):517–26.

40. Perino MT, Yu Q, Myers MJ, et al. Attention alterations in pediatric anxiety: evidence from behavior and neuroimaging. Biol Psychiatry 2021;89(7):726–34.

41. Strawn JR, Bitter SM, Weber WA, et al. Neurocircuitry of generalized anxiety disorder in adolescents: a pilot functional neuroimaging and functional connectivity study. Depress Anxiety 2012;29(11):939–47.

42. Dobson ET, Croarkin PE, Schroeder HK, et al. Bridging anxiety and depression: a network approach in anxious adolescents. J Affect Disord 2021;280(Pt A): 305–14.

43. Walkup JT, Friedland SJ, Peris TS, et al. Dysregulation, catastrophic reactions, and the anxiety disorders. Child Adolesc Psychiatr Clin N Am 2021;30(2): 431–44.

44. Fjermestad KW, Lium C, Heiervang ER, et al. Parental internalizing symptoms as predictors of anxiety symptoms in clinic-referred children. Scand J Child Adolesc Psychiatr Psychol 2020;8:18–24.

45. Strawn JR, Lu L, Peris TS, et al. Research review: pediatric anxiety disorders - what have we learnt in the last 10 years? J Child Psychol Psychiatry 2021;62(2): 114–39.

46. Beesdo K, Pine DS, Lieb R, et al. Incidence and risk patterns of anxiety and depressive disorders and categorization of generalized anxiety disorder. Arch Gen Psychiatry 2010;67(1):47–57.

47. Casline E, Patel ZS, Timpano KR, et al. Exploring the link between transdiagnostic cognitive risk factors, anxiogenic parenting behaviors, and child anxiety. Child Psychiatry Hum Dev 2021;52(6):1032–43.

48. Cote SM, Ahun MN, Herba CM, et al. Why is maternal depression related to adolescent internalizing problems? a 15-year population-based study. J Am Acad Child Adolesc Psychiatry 2018;57(12):916–24.

49. Grabow AP, Khurana A, Natsuaki MN, et al. Using an adoption-biological family design to examine associations between maternal trauma, maternal depressive symptoms, and child internalizing and externalizing behaviors. Dev Psychopathol 2017;29(5):1707–20.

50. Hails KA, Reuben JD, Shaw DS, et al. Transactional associations among maternal depression, parent-child coercion, and child conduct problems during early childhood. J Clin Child Adolesc Psychol 2018;47(sup1):S291–305.

51. Volling BL, Yu T, Gonzalez R, et al. Maternal and paternal trajectories of depressive symptoms predict family risk and children's emotional and behavioral problems after the birth of a sibling. Dev Psychopathol 2019;31(4):1307–24.

52. Mina K, Dulcan RRB, Poonam JHA, et al. Children of psychiatrically ill parents: risks and resilience. Concise guide to child & adolescent Psychiatry. 5th Edition. Arlington, VA: American Psychiatric Association Publishing; 2018. p. 297–9.

53. Lieb R, Wittchen HU, Hofler M, et al. Parental psychopathology, parenting styles, and the risk of social phobia in offspring: a prospective-longitudinal community study. Arch Gen Psychiatry 2000;57(9):859–66.

54. Fyer AJ, Mannuzza S, Chapman TF, et al. Specificity in familial aggregation of phobic disorders. Arch Gen Psychiatry 1995;52(7):564–73.

55. Cooper PJ, Fearn V, Willetts L, et al. Affective disorder in the parents of a clinic sample of children with anxiety disorders. J Affect Disord 2006;93(1–3):205–12.

56. Aktar E, Majdandzic M, De Vente W, et al. Parental expressions of anxiety and child temperament in toddlerhood jointly predict preschoolers' avoidance of novelty. J Clin Child Adolesc Psychol 2018;47(sup1):S421–34.

57. Poole KL, Van Lieshout RJ, McHolm AE, et al. Trajectories of social anxiety in children: influence of child cortisol reactivity and parental social anxiety. J Abnorm Child Psychol 2018;46(6):1309–19.

58. Steinsbekk S, Berg-Nielsen TS, Belsky J, et al. Parents' personality-disorder symptoms predict children's symptoms of anxiety and depressive disorders - a prospective cohort study. J Abnorm Child Psychol 2019;47(12):1931–43.

59. Wilson S, Durbin CE. Parental personality disorder symptoms are associated with dysfunctional parent-child interactions during early childhood: a multilevel modeling analysis. Personal Disord 2012;3(1):55–65.

60. Melton TH, Croarkin PE, Strawn JR, et al. Comorbid anxiety and depressive symptoms in children and adolescents: a systematic review and analysis. J Psychiatr Pract 2016;22(2):84–98.

61. Turgeon L, O'Connor KP, Marchand A, et al. Recollections of parent-child relationships in patients with obsessive-compulsive disorder and panic disorder with agoraphobia. Acta Psychiatr Scand 2002;105(4):310–6.

62. Yap MB, Pilkington PD, Ryan SM, et al. Parental factors associated with depression and anxiety in young people: a systematic review and meta-analysis. J Affect Disord 2014;156:8–23.

63. Ollendick TH, Grills AE. Perceived control, family environment, and the etiology of child anxiety-revisited. Behav Ther 2016;47(5):633–42.

64. Affrunti NW, Ginsburg GS. Exploring parental predictors of child anxiety: the mediating role of child interpretation bias. Child Youth Care Forum 2012;41(6):517–27.

65. Lo BCY, Chan SK, Ng TK, et al. Parental demandingness and executive functioning in predicting anxiety among children in a longitudinal community study. J Youth Adolesc 2020;49(1):299–310.
66. Hudson JL, Dodd HF, Bovopoulos N. Temperament, family environment and anxiety in preschool children. J Abnorm Child Psychol 2011;39(7):939–51.
67. Shamir-Essakow G, Ungerer JA, Rapee RM. Attachment, behavioral inhibition, and anxiety in preschool children. J Abnorm Child Psychol 2005;33(2):131–43.
68. Wagner NJ, Gueron-Sela N, Bedford R, et al. Maternal attributions of infant behavior and parenting in toddlerhood predict teacher-rated internalizing problems in childhood. J Clin Child Adolesc Psychol 2018;47(sup1):S569–77.
69. Mak HW, Iacovou M. Dimensions of the parent-child relationship: effects on substance use in adolescence and adulthood. Subst Use Misuse 2019;54(5): 724–36.
70. Bakhla AK, Sinha P, Sharan R, et al. Anxiety in school students: role of parenting and gender. Ind Psychiatry J 2013;22(2):131–7.
71. Fransson M, Granqvist P, Marciszko C, et al. Is middle childhood attachment related to social functioning in young adulthood? Scand J Psychol 2016;57(2): 108–16.
72. Groh AM, Fearon RP, Bakermans-Kranenburg MJ, et al. The significance of attachment security for children's social competence with peers: a meta-analytic study. Attach Hum Dev 2014;16(2):103–36.
73. Bowlby J. Attachment theory and its therapeutic implications. Adolesc Psychiatry 1978;6:5–33.
74. Manassis K, Bradley S, Goldberg S, et al. Behavioural inhibition, attachment and anxiety in children of mothers with anxiety disorders. Can J Psychiatry 1995; 40(2):87–92.
75. Bogels SM, Brechman-Toussaint ML. Family issues in child anxiety: attachment, family functioning, parental rearing and beliefs. Clin Psychol Rev 2006;26(7): 834–56.
76. Colonnesi C, Draijer EM, Jan JMSG, et al. The relation between insecure attachment and child anxiety: a meta-analytic review. J Clin Child Adolesc Psychol 2011;40(4):630–45.
77. Lewis-Morrarty E, Degnan KA, Chronis-Tuscano A, et al. Infant attachment security and early childhood behavioral inhibition interact to predict adolescent social anxiety symptoms. Child Dev 2015;86(2):598–613.
78. Kessler RC, McLaughlin KA, Green JG, et al. Childhood adversities and adult psychopathology in the WHO world mental health surveys. Br J Psychiatry 2010;197(5):378–85.
79. Elmore AL, Crouch E. The association of adverse childhood experiences with anxiety and depression for children and youth, 8 to 17 years of age. Acad Pediatr 2020;20(5):600–8.
80. Karatekin C. Adverse childhood experiences (ACEs), stress and mental health in college students. Stress Health 2018;34(1):36–45.
81. Carr CP, Martins CM, Stingel AM, et al. The role of early life stress in adult psychiatric disorders: a systematic review according to childhood trauma subtypes. J Nerv Ment Dis 2013;201(12):1007–20.
82. Juruena MF, Eror F, Cleare AJ, et al. The role of early life stress in HPA Axis and anxiety. Adv Exp Med Biol 2020;1191:141–53.
83. Schilling C, Weidner K, Schellong J, et al. Patterns of childhood abuse and neglect as predictors of treatment outcome in inpatient psychotherapy: a typological approach. Psychopathology 2015;48(2):91–100.

84. Chorpita BF, Barlow DH. The development of anxiety: the role of control in the early environment. Psychol Bull 1998;124(1):3–21.
85. Hudson JL, Rapee RM. Parent-child interactions and anxiety disorders: an observational study. Behav Res Ther 2001;39(12):1411–27.
86. Allen JL, Rapee RM, Sandberg S. Severe life events and chronic adversities as antecedents to anxiety in children: a matched control study. J Abnorm Child Psychol 2008;36(7):1047–56.
87. Boer F, Markus MT, Maingay R, et al. Negative life events of anxiety disordered children: bad fortune, vulnerability, or reporter bias? Child Psychiatry Hum Dev Spring 2002;32(3):187–99.
88. Gothelf D, Aharonovsky O, Horesh N, et al. Life events and personality factors in children and adolescents with obsessive-compulsive disorder and other anxiety disorders. Compr Psychiatry 2004;45(3):192–8.
89. Draisey J, Halldorsson B, Cooper P, et al. Associations between family factors, childhood adversity, negative life events and child anxiety disorders: an exploratory study of diagnostic specificity. Behav Cogn Psychother 2020;48(3): 253–67.
90. Kalin NH. Anxiety, depression, and suicide in youth. Am J Psychiatry 2021; 178(4):275–9.
91. Rudenstine S, McNeal K, Schulder T, et al. Depression and anxiety during the COVID-19 pandemic in an urban, low-income public university sample. J Trauma Stress 2021;34(1):12–22.
92. Miller GE, White SF, Chen E, et al. Association of Inflammatory activity with larger neural responses to threat and reward among children living in poverty. Am J Psychiatry 2021;178(4):313–20.
93. Modecki KL, Minchin J, Harbaugh AG, et al. Bullying prevalence across contexts: a meta-analysis measuring cyber and traditional bullying. J Adolesc Health 2014;55(5):602–11.
94. McKay MT, Cannon M, Chambers D, et al. Childhood trauma and adult mental disorder: a systematic review and meta-analysis of longitudinal cohort studies. Acta Psychiatr Scand 2021;143(3):189–205.
95. Takizawa R, Maughan B, Arseneault L. Adult health outcomes of childhood bullying victimization: evidence from a five-decade longitudinal British birth cohort. Am J Psychiatry 2014;171(7):777–84.
96. Rose CA, Tynes BM. Longitudinal associations between cybervictimization and mental health among U.S. Adolescents. J Adolesc Health 2015;57(3):305–12.
97. Merikangas KR, He JP, Brody D, et al. Prevalence and treatment of mental disorders among US children in the 2001-2004 NHANES. Pediatrics 2010;125(1): 75–81.
98. Nock MK, Kazdin AE, Hiripi E, et al. Lifetime prevalence, correlates, and persistence of oppositional defiant disorder: results from the National Comorbidity Survey Replication. J Child Psychol Psychiatry 2007;48(7):703–13.
99. Beesdo K, Knappe S, Pine DS. Anxiety and anxiety disorders in children and adolescents: developmental issues and implications for DSM-V. Psychiatr Clin North Am 2009;32(3):483–524.
100. Knappe S, Martini J, Muris P, et al. Progression of externalizing disorders into anxiety disorders: longitudinal transitions in the first three decades of life. J Anxiety Disord 2022;86:102533.
101. Wichstrom L, Belsky J, Steinsbekk S. Homotypic and heterotypic continuity of symptoms of psychiatric disorders from age 4 to 10 years: a dynamic panel model. J Child Psychol Psychiatry 2017;58(11):1239–47.

102. Michelini G, Eley TC, Gregory AM, et al. Aetiological overlap between anxiety and attention deficit hyperactivity symptom dimensions in adolescence. J Child Psychol Psychiatry 2015;56(4):423–31.
103. Mogg K, Salum GA, Bradley BP, et al. Attention network functioning in children with anxiety disorders, attention-deficit/hyperactivity disorder and non-clinical anxiety. Psychol Med 2015;45(12):2633–46.
104. Stenseng F, Belsky J, Skalicka V, et al. Peer rejection and attention deficit hyperactivity disorder symptoms: reciprocal relations through ages 4, 6, and 8. Child Dev 2016;87(2):365–73.
105. Wichstrom L, Belsky J, Berg-Nielsen TS. Preschool predictors of childhood anxiety disorders: a prospective community study. J Child Psychol Psychiatry 2013; 54(12):1327–36.
106. Jackson ML, Sztendur EM, Diamond NT, et al. Sleep difficulties and the development of depression and anxiety: a longitudinal study of young Australian women. Arch Womens Ment Health 2014;17(3):189–98.
107. Gregory AM, Caspi A, Eley TC, et al. Prospective longitudinal associations between persistent sleep problems in childhood and anxiety and depression disorders in adulthood. J Abnorm Child Psychol 2005;33(2):157–63.
108. Meijer AM, Reitz E, Dekovic M, et al. Longitudinal relations between sleep quality, time in bed and adolescent problem behaviour. J Child Psychol Psychiatry 2010;51(11):1278–86.
109. Shanahan L, Copeland WE, Angold A, et al. Sleep problems predict and are predicted by generalized anxiety/depression and oppositional defiant disorder. J Am Acad Child Adolesc Psychiatry 2014;53(5):550–8.
110. Yoo SS, Gujar N, Hu P, et al. The human emotional brain without sleep–a prefrontal amygdala disconnect. Curr Biol 2007;17(20):R877–8.
111. McGowan SK, Behar E, Luhmann M. Examining the relationship between worry and sleep: a daily process approach. Behav Ther 2016;47(4):460–73.
112. Bai S, Ricketts EJ, Thamrin H, et al. Longitudinal study of sleep and internalizing problems in youth treated for pediatric anxiety disorders. J Abnorm Child Psychol 2020;48(1):67–77.
113. Kelly RJ, El-Sheikh M. Reciprocal relations between children's sleep and their adjustment over time. Dev Psychol 2014;50(4):1137–47.
114. Zimmermann P, Wittchen HU, Hofler M, et al. Primary anxiety disorders and the development of subsequent alcohol use disorders: a 4-year community study of adolescents and young adults. Psychol Med 2003;33(7):1211–22.
115. Mathew AR, Norton PJ, Zvolensky MJ, et al. Smoking behavior and alcohol consumption in individuals with panic attacks. J Cogn Psychother 2011;25(1): 61–70.
116. Blumenthal H, Cloutier RM, Zamboanga BL, et al. A laboratory-based test of the relation between adolescent alcohol use and panic-relevant responding. Exp Clin Psychopharmacol 2015;23(5):303–13.
117. Nixon K, McClain JA. Adolescence as a critical window for developing an alcohol use disorder: current findings in neuroscience. Curr Opin Psychiatry 2010;23(3):227–32.
118. Allan CA. Alcohol problems and anxiety disorders–a critical review. Alcohol Alcohol 1995;30(2):145–51.
119. Pandey SC, Sakharkar AJ, Tang L, et al. Potential role of adolescent alcohol exposure-induced amygdaloid histone modifications in anxiety and alcohol intake during adulthood. Neurobiol Dis 2015;82:607–19.

120. Pascual M, Do Couto BR, Alfonso-Loeches S, et al. Changes in histone acetylation in the prefrontal cortex of ethanol-exposed adolescent rats are associated with ethanol-induced place conditioning. Neuropharmacology 2012;62(7): 2309–19.

121. Goodwin RD, Gotlib IH. Panic attacks and psychopathology among youth. Acta Psychiatr Scand 2004;109(3):216–21.

122. Degenhardt L, Coffey C, Romaniuk H, et al. The persistence of the association between adolescent cannabis use and common mental disorders into young adulthood. Addiction 2013;108(1):124–33.

123. Zhang C, Ye M, Fu Y, et al. The psychological impact of the COVID-19 pandemic on teenagers in China. J Adolesc Health 2020;67(6):747–55.

124. Jones EAK, Mitra AK, Bhuiyan AR. Impact of COVID-19 on mental health in adolescents: a systematic review. Int J Environ Res Public Health 2021;18(5). https://doi.org/10.3390/ijerph18052470.

125. Sinha R. Chronic stress, drug use, and vulnerability to addiction. Ann N Y Acad Sci 2008;1141:105–30.

126. Brokamp C, Strawn JR, Beck AF, et al. Pediatric psychiatric emergency department utilization and fine particulate matter: a case-crossover study. Environ Health Perspect 2019;127(9):97006.

127. Brunst KJ, Ryan PH, Altaye M, et al. Myo-inositol mediates the effects of traffic-related air pollution on generalized anxiety symptoms at age 12years. Environ Res 2019;175:71–8.

128. Patel NB, Xu Y, McCandless LC, et al. Very low-level prenatal mercury exposure and behaviors in children: the HOME Study. Environ Health 2019;18(1):4.

129. Gavin B, Lyne J, McNicholas F. Mental health and the COVID-19 pandemic. Ir J Psychol Med 2020;37(3):156–8.

130. Racine N, McArthur BA, Cooke JE, et al. Global prevalence of depressive and anxiety symptoms in children and adolescents during COVID-19: a meta-analysis. JAMA Pediatr 2021;175(11):1142–50.

131. Qi M, Zhou SJ, Guo ZC, et al. The effect of social support on mental health in Chinese adolescents during the outbreak of COVID-19. J Adolesc Health 2020;67(4):514–8.

132. Masonbrink AR, Hurley E. Advocating for children during the COVID-19 school closures. Pediatrics 2020;146(3). https://doi.org/10.1542/peds.2020-1440.

133. Goodwin RD. Association between infection early in life and mental disorders among youth in the community: a cross-sectional study. BMC Public Health 2011;11:878.

134. Wu Y, Xu X, Chen Z, et al. Nervous system involvement after infection with COVID-19 and other coronaviruses. Brain Behav Immun 2020;87:18–22.

135. Desforges M, Le Coupanec A, Dubeau P, et al. Human coronaviruses and other respiratory viruses: underestimated opportunistic pathogens of the central nervous system? Viruses 2019;12(1). https://doi.org/10.3390/v12010014.

136. Dantzer R. Neuroimmune interactions: from the brain to the immune system and vice versa. Physiol Rev 2018;98(1):477–504.

137. Hu Y, Chen Y, Zheng Y, et al. Factors related to mental health of inpatients with COVID-19 in Wuhan, China. Brain Behav Immun 2020;89:587–93.

138. Ahmad SJ, Feigen CM, Vazquez JP, et al. Neurological sequelae of COVID-19. J Integr Neurosci 2022;21(3):77.

139. Howe AS, Buttenschon HN, Bani-Fatemi A, et al. Candidate genes in panic disorder: meta-analyses of 23 common variants in major anxiogenic pathways. Mol Psychiatry 2016;21(5):665–79.

140. Levey DF, Gelernter J, Polimanti R, et al. Reproducible genetic risk loci for anxiety: results from approximately 200,000 participants in the million veteran program. Am J Psychiatry 2020;177(3):223–32.

141. Chawner S, Owen MJ, Holmans P, et al. Genotype-phenotype associations in children with copy number variants associated with high neuropsychiatric risk in the UK (IMAGINE-ID): a case-control cohort study. Lancet Psychiatry 2019; 6(6):493–505.

142. Penninx BW, Pine DS, Holmes EA, et al. Anxiety disorders. Lancet 2021; 397(10277):914–27.

143. Maron E, Nutt D. Biological markers of generalized anxiety disorder. Dialogues Clin Neurosci 2017;19(2):147–58.

144. Tadic A, Rujescu D, Szegedi A, et al. Association of a MAOA gene variant with generalized anxiety disorder, but not with panic disorder or major depression. Am J Med Genet B Neuropsychiatr Genet 2003;117B(1):1–6.

145. You JS, Hu SY, Chen B, et al. Serotonin transporter and tryptophan hydroxylase gene polymorphisms in Chinese patients with generalized anxiety disorder. Psychiatr Genet 2005;15(1):7–11.

146. Molina E, Cervilla J, Rivera M, et al. Polymorphic variation at the serotonin 1-A receptor gene is associated with comorbid depression and generalized anxiety. Psychiatr Genet 2011;21(4):195–201.

147. Moreira FP, Fabiao JD, Bittencourt G, et al. The Met allele of BDNF Val66Met polymorphism is associated with increased BDNF levels in generalized anxiety disorder. Psychiatr Genet 2015;25(5):201–7.

148. Wang Y, Zhang H, Li Y, et al. BDNF Val66Met polymorphism and plasma levels in Chinese Han population with obsessive-compulsive disorder and generalized anxiety disorder. J Affect Disord 2015;186:7–12.

149. Wingo AP, Gibson G. Blood gene expression profiles suggest altered immune function associated with symptoms of generalized anxiety disorder. Brain Behav Immun 2015;43:184–91.

150. Maron E, Hettema JM, Shlik J. Advances in molecular genetics of panic disorder. Mol Psychiatry 2010;15(7):681–701.

151. Maron E, Lan CC, Nutt D. Imaging and genetic approaches to inform biomarkers for anxiety disorders, obsessive-compulsive disorders, and PSTD. Curr Top Behav Neurosci 2018;40:219–92.

152. Ziegler C, Richter J, Mahr M, et al. MAOA gene hypomethylation in panic disorder-reversibility of an epigenetic risk pattern by psychotherapy. Transl Psychiatry 2016;6:e773.

153. Schartner C, Ziegler C, Schiele MA, et al. CRHR1 promoter hypomethylation: an epigenetic readout of panic disorder? Eur Neuropsychopharmacol 2017;27(4): 360–71.

154. Ziegler C, Dannlowski U, Brauer D, et al. Oxytocin receptor gene methylation: converging multilevel evidence for a role in social anxiety. Neuropsychopharmacology 2015;40(6):1528–38.

155. Samochowiec J, Hajduk A, Samochowiec A, et al. Association studies of MAO-A, COMT, and 5-HTT genes polymorphisms in patients with anxiety disorders of the phobic spectrum. Psychiatry Res 2004;128(1):21–6.

156. Xie B, Wang B, Suo P, et al. Genetic association between BDNF gene polymorphisms and phobic disorders: a case-control study among mainland Han Chinese. J Affect Disord 2011;132(1–2):239–42.

157. Van Houtem CM, Laine ML, Boomsma DI, et al. A review and meta-analysis of the heritability of specific phobia subtypes and corresponding fears. J Anxiety Disord 2013;27(4):379–88.

158. Gelernter J, Page GP, Stein MB, et al. Genome-wide linkage scan for loci predisposing to social phobia: evidence for a chromosome 16 risk locus. Am J Psychiatry 2004;161(1):59–66.

# Developmental Epidemiology of Pediatric Anxiety Disorders

Emily N. Warner, MD, MPH[a,b,*], Robert T. Ammerman, PhD[c],
Tracy A. Glauser, MD[d], John P. Pestian, PhD[d],
Greeshma Agasthya, PhD[e], Jeffrey R. Strawn, MD[a,f,g]

## KEYWORDS

- Anxiety • Prevalence • COVID-19 • Onset • Stability • Recurrence • Remission
- Artificial intelligence

## KEY POINTS

- Anxiety disorders emerge in childhood and are among the most common psychiatric disorders in children and adolescents.
- Anxiety disorders are associated with homotypic continuity and heterotypic continuity.
- Predictors of recurrence in anxiety disorders include traumatic and adverse life events, negative family interactions, adolescent-onset anxiety disorders, and specific demographic characteristics.
- During the COVID-19 pandemic, the prevalence of pediatric anxiety disorders increased, and many youth with anxiety disorders experienced worsening symptoms.

## INTRODUCTION

The core risk phase for the emergence of anxiety occurs between the period of childhood through adolescence. Anxiety symptoms during this phase may range from transient mild to more severe and persistent anxiety disorders. From a clinical and public health perspective, understanding the prevalence, incidence, and longitudinal course

[a] University of Cincinnati College of Medicine, Cincinnati, OH, USA; [b] Department of Environmental and Public Health Sciences, University of Cincinnati; [c] Division of Behavioral Medicine and Clinical Psychology, Department of Pediatrics, Cincinnati Children's Hospital Medical Center, Cincinnati, OH, USA; [d] Department of Pediatrics, Cincinnati Children's Hospital Medical Center, Cincinnati, OH, USA; [e] Oak Ridge National Laboratory, Computational Sciences and Engineering Division, Advanced Computing for Health Sciences Section; [f] Division of Psychiatry, Department of Pediatrics, Cincinnati Children's Hospital Medical Center, Cincinnati, OH, USA; [g] Division of Clinical Pharmacology, Department of Pediatrics, Cincinnati Children's Hospital Medical Center, Cincinnati, OH, USA
* Corresponding author. Department of Psychiatry & Behavioral Neuroscience, University of Cincinnati, Box 670559, 260 Stetson Street, Suite 3200, Cincinnati, OH 45267-0559.
*E-mail address:* warnerey@mail.uc.edu

Child Adolesc Psychiatric Clin N Am 32 (2023) 511–530
https://doi.org/10.1016/j.chc.2023.02.001
1056-4993/23/© 2023 Elsevier Inc. All rights reserved.

**childpsych.theclinics.com**

of anxiety disorders is critical to developing early identification and intervention strategies. COVID-19 has significantly altered the incidence and prevalence of anxiety disorders among youth and may have affected the course of anxiety among those who had already developed anxiety disorders before the pandemic. Of note, the US Preventive Services Task Force (USPSTF) recently updated their guidelines to include screening for anxiety symptoms in children and adolescents ages 8 to 18 years (B recommendation), given the high prevalence of these disorders. A moderate net benefit was found for screening in this age group, with significant benefits for early detection and treatment of anxiety symptoms.[1] The benefit of screening and early treatment was explored within the Evidence Report,[2] but the specific guidance for how screening should occur was not provided. Current evidence supports the implementation of screening and treatment of anxiety disorders in the pediatric primary care setting and evaluating for family history of anxiety disorders early in a child's life as part of routine pediatric care.[3] Further, predictors for recurrence and remission of anxiety disorders are essential for understanding course patterns and improving early recognition, prevention, and treatment strategies across this group.

Anxiety—a normal and basic emotion—is best viewed on a continuum ranging from expected and proportional reactions to environmental factors, novel situations, and everyday challenges to more severe, pathologic forms associated with functional impairment. Excessive anxiety that is "out of proportion" to environmental factors produces avoidance and impairment.[4] Anxiety can be acutely distressing or typically transient and varies across development, even in pathologic forms. Additionally, with anxiety disorders, symptoms persist and can remain into adolescence and/or differentiate into other anxiety disorders throughout childhood and into adulthood. For example, a child with a separation anxiety disorder may develop social and generalized anxiety disorders (GAD) as an adolescent. This article reviews the developmental epidemiology of childhood and adolescent anxiety disorders, considering COVID-19, sex differences, longitudinal course, and stability.

## ONSET OF ANXIETY DISORDERS

Anxiety disorders are among the most common mental illnesses in children and adolescents and have the earliest onset of psychiatric disorders.[5,6] They often begin in childhood and most commonly precede the onset of depression, with a median age of onset around 6 and 13 years, respectively, for each disorder.[6,7]

### Onset and Trajectory of Specific Anxiety Disorders

There is a trend in the onset and temporal course of pediatric anxiety disorders as they often begin as a singular disorder, such as specific phobia, and can develop across a complex trajectory as they emerge into different forms over time. Specific phobia and separation anxiety disorder are found to be most prevalent in early (up to 6 years) and middle childhood (6–8 years),[8] particularly phobia of animals, blood injection injury, and environmental type,[9] with most cases emerging before the age of 12.[10] Separation anxiety disorder typically emerges slightly after a specific phobia with a mean age of onset of 8 years.[11] As children enter middle school (ages 8–12 years), social anxiety disorder often emerges as children become more self-conscious and experience intense anxiety in social situations as they fear negative evaluation from peers.[8,12] Lastly, GAD is found to be the most prevalent disorder from adolescence onward.[8,10]

The Early Developmental Stages of Psychopathology (EDSP) study (N = 3021), launched in 1994, was a prospective longitudinal study in Munich, Germany, of adolescents and young adults (ages 14–24) to study the prevalence and natural course of psychiatric disorders.[13] As shown in **Fig. 1**, the cumulative age of onset distribution for specific types of anxiety disorders in this age group differs substantially from early childhood to adolescence.[14] Consistent with earlier prospective studies,[8] separation anxiety and specific phobia revealed the earliest onset, with roughly 50% of cases emerging before ages 5 and 8 years, respectively. Social anxiety increases in early adolescence, followed by agoraphobia, panic disorder, and GAD, suggesting that late adolescence is a critical period for the emergence of these disorders. Additionally, despite differences in prevalence in EDSP, no significant sex differences were seen in onset patterns.[13]

## PREVALENCE OF ANXIETY DISORDERS

Anxiety disorders are a leading cause of years lived with disability for children and adolescents and, globally, account for 1% of total disability-adjusted life years (DALYs)[15] and have a lifetime prevalence in western countries of 15% to 20%.[16] In the United States, among adolescents aged 13 to 18, the lifetime prevalence of anxiety disorders is 40%.[17] More recently, rates of anxiety disorders among 9- and 12-year-olds are roughly 22%,[5] although collectively, these rates may vary due to methodology. Nonetheless, there is clear evidence that, across the age span, these disorders are highly prevalent. Additionally, the prevalence of anxiety and potential anxiety disorders among adolescents after the onset of the COVID-19 pandemic has nearly doubled compared with pre-pandemic estimates.[18]

### Prevalence Among Anxiety Disorder Type

The most frequent anxiety disorders in children and adolescents include separation anxiety disorder, with prevalence ranging from 3% to 8%; specific phobia, with rates of approximately 15%; and social anxiety disorders, with rates up to 10%.[6,14] More recently, 1 in 10 children were found to have an anxiety disorder at least once among a sample of children between the ages of 4 and 14.[8] Specific phobia and GAD were the most prevalent anxiety disorders, and both increased with age. However, other disorders (eg, panic disorder and social anxiety disorder) also appear to increase with age in different samples.[6] Overall, GAD is the most prevalent disorder among adolescents and young adults.[8,19] In the recent Great Smoky Mountain Study, a longitudinal child epidemiological study that began in 1992 to evaluate the need for mental health services in a rural area of the United States, specific prevalence rates based on age for certain disorders were identified. This included the prevalence of separation anxiety in 9- to 12-year-olds (4–5%)[19] and social anxiety in 4- to 17-year-olds (2.3%).[20] These data highlight the pattern of childhood-onset anxiety disorders that ultimately predict poor mental health outcomes as children progress through adolescence into adulthood. Reduction in childhood distress and early identification and treatment of these specific disorders can help improve anxiety symptoms and disorders among children and adults.

### Biological Sex and Anxiety Disorder Prevalence

Across studies, women have a higher lifetime prevalence of anxiety disorders compared with men,[21] although this difference does not emerge until adolescence. This pattern of emergence is displayed in **Fig. 2**, which reveals a broad depiction of the overall trend regarding the age of onset of anxiety disorders as well as the prevalence difference between sexes during childhood and adolescence. Notably, during early adolescence (age 14), girls become more likely than boys to have generalized

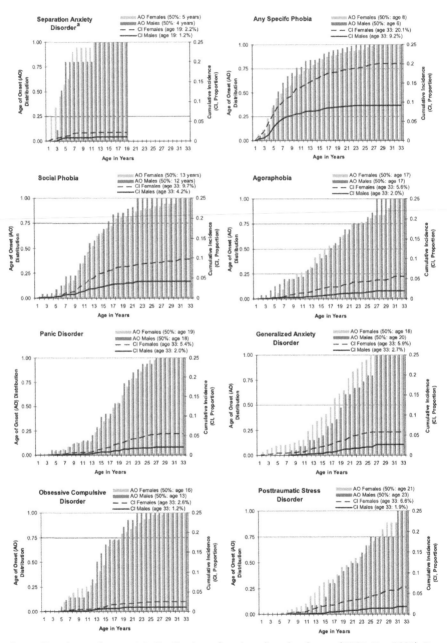

**Fig. 1.** CI and age of onset AO distribution of anxiety disorders by sex (EDSP; N = 3021). Bars show the cumulative age of onset distribution; lines show the age-dependent cumulative lifetime incidence; in phobias, impairment was required among subjects aged 18 years or older. [a]Separation anxiety disorder was only assessed in the younger study cohort. (Katja Beesdo-Baum, Susanne Knappe, Developmental Epidemiology of Anxiety Disorders, Child and Adolescent Psychiatric Clinics of North America, 21 (3), 2012, 457-478, https://doi.org/10.1016/j.chc.2012.05.001.s)

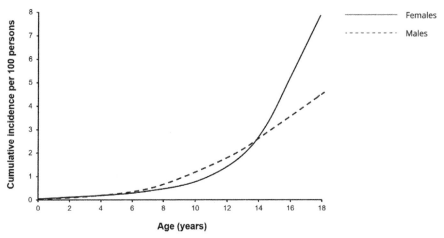

**Fig. 2.** Cumulative incidence per 100 persons of the age of onset of anxiety disorders from ages 0 to 18 years by sex. (*Data adapted from* JAMA Psychiatry (2020): Incidence Rates and Cumulative Incidences of the Full Spectrum of Diagnosed Mental Disorders in Childhood and Adolescence (Dalsgaard et al., 2020).[100])

and social anxiety disorders and specific phobias. During early adolescence, GAD is nearly three times higher in girls than boys.[6] However, before adolescence, sex differences in prevalence rates are small or undetectable, a finding that is consistent with several studies observing sex differences in early adolescence around ages 13 and 15.[22,23] Importantly, why the anxiety disorders are more common in girls than boys and why this difference emerges during puberty is unclear. Biological (puberty), psychological (emotional regulation capacity), and social (internalized gender roles) factors may contribute; however, further investigation is needed, and the cause is likely multifactorial.

### COVID-19 and the Prevalence of Anxiety Disorders in Youth

Prior to the COVID-19 pandemic, rates of clinically significant GAD in large youth cohorts were approximately 12%.[24] Concerningly, recent meta-analyses of the global prevalence of anxiety disorders in children and adolescents during COVID-19 suggest that the rate of clinically elevated anxiety among youth is approximately 20%.[18] Cross-sectional studies, including those by Duan and colleagues,[25] have found similar increases in significant anxiety in children and adolescents in China during the epidemic.[26] In this sample, the pandemic was associated with increased prevalence in five anxiety dimensions: separation anxiety, fear of physical injury, social anxiety, panic disorder, and generalized anxiety. Further, a parent–child discussion was a protective factor; children and adolescents who discussed the pandemic with their parents have fewer anxiety symptoms,[27] raising the possibility that intolerance of uncertainty or uncertainty itself, as well as family environment, significantly affects the risk of developing anxiety, particularly during times of stress/crisis.[28] Intolerance of uncertainty involves a set of negative beliefs about unfamiliar situations and leads to avoidance of uncertain situations and more significant anxiety symptoms in youth. The COVID-19 pandemic was an unfamiliar and anxiety-provoking situation for both children and adults, with open communication and "warm" familial environments serving as protective factors for worsening anxiety symptoms during this time.[29,30]

Clinically significant anxiety among children and adolescents appears to be increasing since the COVID-19 pandemic. However, to date, most studies are cross-sectional and provide a single-time snapshot rather than a true longitudinal glimpse into the temporal course of these anxiety symptoms or anxiety disorders. Whether these patterns reflect transient perturbations, adjustment-type reactions, or the true development of enduring anxiety disorders remains to be determined.

### Longitudinal Impact of COVID-19 on Anxiety Prevalence

In our recent longitudinal studies of adolescents aged 12 to 17 years with primary anxiety disorders,[31] adolescents with laboratory-confirmed Severe Acute Respiratory Syndrome Coronavirus-2 (SARS-CoV-2) infection, anxiety symptoms among adolescents significantly worsened for most specific anxiety symptoms, based on the GAD-7[32] scale that was administered weekly. In addition, clinical severity—reflected by Clinical Global Impression-Severity (CGI-S) scores—significantly worsened. Also, central nervous system (CNS) post-acute sequelae SARS-CoV-2 infection (PASC) symptoms (hypersomnia, irritability, concentration, motivation/involvement, and energy) generally worsened in these anxious adolescents following SARS-CoV-2 infection. Further, and of clinical significance, COVID-19 was associated with a 33% worsening in anxiety. These data highlight the possibility that COVID-19 is associated with a wide array of neuropsychiatric symptoms among anxious youth. Further investigation into the interplay of neurotropic, inflammatory, and psychosocial factors of SARS-CoV-2 is needed.

## LONGITUDINAL COURSE

Anxiety disorders wax and wane over time, and their persistence is primarily due to recurrence rather than chronic symptoms.[14] Although childhood-onset anxiety disorders may spontaneously remit, they are generally persistent.[33] However, "syndrome shift" to other disorders is common. These processes, as well as disorder "stability" are generally categorized as follows.

- *Homotypic continuity:* the same anxiety disorder remains present later in life. For example, a 9-year-old child with social anxiety disorder continues to meet syndromic criteria for a social anxiety disorder at age 13 and age 17.
- *Heterotypic continuity:* an anxiety disorder shifts to a different diagnosis. For example, a young adolescent with a GAD at age 13 develops a substance use disorder or major depressive disorder in late adolescence.

Population-based data suggest that, for anxiety disorders, homotypic continuity is more common than heterotypic continuity from adolescence to adulthood.[34,35] Specifically, homotypic continuity has been observed for social anxiety disorder, simple phobia, and GAD.[36] In contrast, heterotypic continuity depends on developmental phases. For example, in early childhood, anxiety disorders generally precede depression,[37] while from adolescence to adulthood, anxiety and depression can cross-predict one another (i.e., anxiety follows depression and vice versa).[38] Additionally, anxiety disorders in adulthood exhibit little homotypic continuity from adolescence but instead are precipitated by depression.[39] This finding has important implications when one considers patients with major depressive disorders with anxious distress or major depressive disorder with a co-occurring anxiety disorder in that several studies suggest that the presence of co-occurring anxiety—regardless of whether it came first or second—decreases treatment response and increases morbidity and suicide attempts.[19] For example, in children aged 9 to 16 years within the Great Smoky

Mountain Study, the risk for suicidal ideation was greatest in subjects with overlapping depression plus anxiety.[40,41] Additionally, disentangling true comorbidity from syndromic overlap is difficult, particularly for children and adolescents with anxiety disorders. For example, children or adolescents with anxiety disorders frequently experience irritability and avoidance. These symptoms can be confused with symptoms of depression—irritability and withdrawal/disinterest. As anxiety symptoms persist, youth may experience demoralization and frustration, which can precipitate feelings of "sadness" and episodes of tearfulness and guilt, which may again be mistaken for symptoms of a depressive disorder.[3] This further reinforces the need for the updated USPSTF screening recommendations for anxiety-specific mental health screening in children, as many anxiety disorders can be mischaracterized through symptom overlap, such as the case of anxiety-related demoralization misdiagnosed as depression.[3]

Different trajectories of broad anxiety across age groups have been demonstrated, with specific developmental periods linked to dimension-specific symptoms.[42] Broad anxiety, in this sense, is defined as a dysregulation of the anxiety-response system along with resulting distress and impairment, both of which are core features of maladaptive anxiety.[43] For example, children with high levels of broad anxiety experience more separation anxiety symptoms earlier, but these improved with age—however, similar levels of generalized and social anxiety increase over time. Children with high levels of broad anxiety exhibit dysregulation of fear and anxiety-response systems and, as a result, are less able to cope with normative developmental challenges.[42,43] These findings support the notion that development- and age-specific anxiety disorders are strongly influenced by developmental stages (ie, separation anxiety as a younger child; social anxiety as children reach adolescence). For example, flexibility of the fear response, including the capacity to express and extinguish fear, undergoes dynamic changes across development. Specifically, adolescence is a developmental stage when anxiety disorders peak, with underlying neuromodulation changes that occur during this time related to fear-based neural circuitry.[44] During adolescence, teenagers display an extinction of cued fear response and suppressed expression of contextual fear, with changes related to structural connectivity in specific brain regions, such as the PFC.[45] In other words, adolescents experience a reduced fear response to external stimuli with corresponding structural brain changes during this developmental period. These findings highlight the adaptive and developmental differences between anxiety disorders that arise for specific age groups, making certain developmental periods more susceptible to anxiety-related symptoms and disorders.

### Separation Anxiety Disorder

Separation anxiety exhibits continuity from early (4–6 years) to middle childhood, although from age 8 to 9 to age 13 to 14, it decreases.[42] That said, more than a third of children with separation anxiety disorder (36%) exhibit a homotypic pattern with persistence into adulthood.[46] Importantly, separation anxiety disorder or severe separation anxiety may predict the onset of other anxiety disorders (i.e., heterotypic continuity). Increased separation anxiety disorder in middle childhood (8–10 years) predicts GAD in adolescence[8] and there is a reciprocal heterotypic relationship between increased separation anxiety disorder and increased GAD from middle childhood to adolescence. Although some individual studies found a later increase in depression among children diagnosed with separation anxiety disorder,[37,47] a separate meta-analysis indicated no overall substantial increase in the risk of later depression.[48] Alternatively, a clear relationship was established between childhood separation anxiety disorder and the development of panic disorder later in life.[48] This is consistent with previous literature from the Virginia Twin Study of Adolescent Behavioral Development (N = 2762), where childhood separation anxiety disorder predicted adult-onset panic attacks.[49] This trend supports the developmental and temporal perspective on anxiety disorders, with common risk factors first leading to stranger anxiety,[50] then separation anxiety, and later panic and other anxiety disorders.[48]

### Specific Phobia

Specific phobia often begins in early childhood with little homotypic continuity throughout the lifespan. Symptoms of specific phobia demonstrated some continuity from early (4–6 years) to middle childhood (8–10 years).[8] However, in general, specific phobia symptoms in early childhood are associated with a heterotypic path and predict GAD symptoms in middle childhood and adolescence, as well as panic disorder and mixed GAD-panic disorders.[51] One proposed theory[42] is that broad anxiety is expressed as more specific phobias or separation anxiety at younger ages. As children age and developmental demands increase (eg, academic stress, social anxiety), this may result in a more generalized characteristic of worrying and anxiety that is not specific to a particular stimulus.[42] The presence of specific phobia as a child may therefore alert parents and clinicians to the risk of more generalized anxiety symptoms in the future, underscoring the importance of understanding the developmental course of early anxiety symptoms with regard to the long-term risk of developing anxiety.

### Social Anxiety Disorder

Social anxiety disorder generally emerges during childhood and adolescence.[52] However, unlike separation anxiety disorder and GAD, which increase in prevalence from preschool to school age, the prevalence of social anxiety disorder remains stable during this period. Then, when children enter middle childhood (ages 8–10), social anxiety increases, particularly in those who have already experienced subsyndromal anxiety.[8,42] This suggests that children with high levels of anxiety across time may be more sensitive to developmentally specific challenges, such as transitioning to middle school and navigating social pressure among peers. Friendships and peer relationships throughout this period become stronger and more complex, leading to difficulty meeting social demands as children may become overwhelmed and exhibit maladaptive anxiety symptoms in social settings.

Social anxiety disorder during adolescence has heterotypic continuity with depression during early adulthood.[53] Similarly, a social anxiety disorder in adolescence has been shown to increase the risk of future substance abuse, including alcohol[54] and cannabis use.[55] Generally, heterotypic continuity is more common than homotypic continuity in social anxiety disorders.[56] Of note, adolescence has been suggested as a period of heightened learning and flexibility.[57] This raises the question of whether adolescence may be an optimal time to target risks associated with social anxiety disorder and prevent other subsequent heterotypic conditions.

### Generalized Anxiety Disorder

GAD increases from preschool to school age, compared to social anxiety and specific phobia.[8] A pattern of homotypic continuity was found for childhood diagnoses of GAD,[51] where children who develop GAD during middle childhood tend continue to have GAD symptoms during adolescence.[8] Additionally, those who develop GAD symptoms during middle childhood also commonly display symptoms of specific phobia and separation anxiety. GAD symptoms in middle childhood predicted separation anxiety disorder in adolescence (and vice versa). It is important to note that

GAD has a strong association with social anxiety disorder, and these disorders often co-occurr and have overlapping features.[58] In contrast to this homotypic trend, GAD in adolescence predicts adult depression.[36,37,59] There is some suggestion that depressive symptoms may be a complication or consequence of untreated and chronic GAD, given the large number of GAD patients who go on to develop major depression and the shared "bridging" symptoms between the two disorders (eg, excessive tearfulness, low self-esteem, impaired schoolwork, appetite changes, and physical symptoms).[60] However, other studies argue against a shared underlying genotype, given each disorder's risk factors.[61] Multiple biological, environmental, and social factors influence this complex relationship between anxiety and depressive symptoms in youth, with the suggestion that these common bridging symptom clusters may play a critical role in the pathogenesis of comorbid depressive disorders among youth with anxiety disorders.[60]

### Panic Disorder

Based on current findings, childhood panic disorder and GAD are among the strongest predictors of developing a panic disorder and/or GAD in adults. Many prior studies have examined anxiety disorders as a whole, displaying homotypic continuity trends, including the homotypic pattern of childhood panic disorder developing into adult panic disorder.[38] These data are supported by Newman and colleagues,[51] who showed a pattern of broad homotypic continuity specifically for participants who developed panic disorder as a child and continued to display symptoms of panic disorder and/or mixed GAD-panic disorder into adulthood. The identification of developmental risk factors, including a childhood diagnosis of panic disorder, may facilitate the prevention of GAD and panic disorder later in adulthood. However, there is significant heterogeneity concerning the phenomenon of panic attacks, and they can accompany any psychiatric disorder. This ubiquity is reflected in the *DSM-5* "with panic attacks" which can be added to any disorder and further underscores the frequency of panic symptoms and raises the possibility of even more etiologic diversity.

## LONGITUDINAL COURSE: SEX

The course—like prevalence—of anxiety disorders is strongly influenced by biological sex. Women are more likely than men to have elevated or increasing levels of anxiety over time.[62] Additionally, women experience more overall impairment, decreased global functioning, and more problems with family life.[63] In the Child/Adolescent Anxiety Multimodal Study (CAMS), young women participants were less likely to be free from anxiety disorders compared with young men 6.5 years post-treatment. Through a descriptive analysis among college students in China, women suffered significantly higher anxiety than men, particularly during their first and second years.[64] This is consistent with studies of sex differences among college students in different contexts showing similar anxiety trends in women.[65,66] Adolescence is a critical period of emerging anxiety among women, underscoring the need for early identification of at-risk adolescents for targeted prevention.

In a double-cohort longitudinal study involving adolescents aged 10 to 20, 91% of participants followed a trajectory of initially low anxiety levels that decreased over time, while 9% followed higher initial anxiety levels that increased over time. Within this study, women were more likely to follow the high-increasing trajectory than men.[67] Similarly, Legerstee and colleagues found that a subgroup of adolescent girls experienced progressively increasing anxiety beginning in mid-adolescence. In contrast, boys had a progressive decrease in anxiety during this period.[68] Further, in this study, the increase in anxiety symptoms during mid-adolescence represented an at-risk anxiety trajectory of individuals who developed psychiatric disorders during adolescence and early adulthood, with 40% of girls in this group having an anxiety disorder. These findings emphasize the importance of a targeted prevention program in early adolescence and the need for early intervention when children begin to experience anxiety in mid-adolescence.[69]

## STABILITY OF ANXIETY DISORDERS

Anxiety symptoms, particularly in early childhood, do not always predict later anxiety symptoms.[8] However, in middle childhood, these symptoms are less likely to remit, which highlights this developmental period as crucial for preventive and treatment efforts. Specific phobia and GAD were the most prevalent anxiety disorders and increased with age, whereas separation anxiety disorder and social anxiety disorders were relatively rare. In early and middle childhood, there was some stability between symptoms observed as well as between middle childhood and adolescence. However, in early childhood and adolescence, there was no continuity between symptoms. Of note, the homotypic stability of anxiety disorders was present in middle childhood but not before this.[5] These findings are consistent with previous studies[37] suggesting that diagnostic remission for a specific type of anxiety disorder does not necessarily mean complete remission as there is significant "mobility" between diagnostic classes.

Within the National Comorbidity Survey-Adolescent Supplement (NCS-A), anxiety disorders were markedly more persistent than mood or substance use disorders, suggesting the enduring nature of these disorders and the difficulty in regard to treatment and remission, compared with other disorders that show susceptibility during this developmental period.[53] Additionally, a multi-generational study showed that children with persistent anxiety disorder trajectory reported a higher proportion of other psychiatric disorders during childhood than those in the non-persistent trajectory.[70] This suggests that children with more persistent anxiety may need increased monitoring and screening for other psychiatric disorders.

### Stability of Anxiety Disorders in Child/Adolescent Anxiety Multimodal Study/Child/Adolescent Anxiety Multimodal Extended Long-Term Study

In the multisite CAMS, 319 anxious youth across four consecutive years were randomized to one of four treatment conditions (cognitive behavioral therapy [CBT], selective serotonin reuptake inhibitors [SSRIs], combination of SSRI and CBT, or pill placebo). The youth then entered the Child/Adolescent Anxiety Multimodal Extended Long-term Study (CAMELS) between 4 and 12 years after initial treatment with either CBT, an SSRI, CBT + SSRI, or placebo and were assessed annually over 5 years.[71] Despite 12 weeks of evidence-based treatment in most patients, just under half of the sample (47%) experienced stable remission 6 years after randomization.[72] This finding can be seen from multiple perspectives. First, it could reflect the chronic nature of pediatric anxiety disorders and underscores the need for enhanced treatment and relapse prevention strategies. Second, the finding could be seen in terms of short-term treatment ($\leq$12 weeks) being inadequate to produce sustained remission and raises questions related to treatment sequencing (psychotherapy before medication or medication before psychotherapy) and treatment combination (eg, CBT + pharmacotherapy). Just over one in five youths were consistently free from all anxiety disorders for the follow-up study. In contrast, the remainder of the youth showed a pattern of relapse or chronic illness with ongoing engagement in mental health treatment services. However, despite the persistence or relapse of the anxiety disorder, treatment decreased the severity of these disorders or, in some other way, prevented the development of secondary pathology remains a possibility. Other cross-sectional studies reveal that CBT and pharmacotherapy (eg, SSRIs) significantly reduce anxiety in the short term[73] but long-term outcomes are less clear.

Youth who significantly improve following short-term treatment (ie, 12 weeks) are more likely to be in stable remission, regardless of whether they received an SSRI, psychotherapy, or the combination.[72] This suggests the long-term benefits of receiving treatment early in the course of these disorders. Additionally, youth who were younger at the start of treatment are more likely to experience stable remission in the long term.

## RECURRENCE AND REMISSION OF ANXIETY DISORDERS IN YOUTH
### Predictors for Recurrence

Overall predictors for the recurrence of anxiety disorders among children and adolescents include family factors, baseline disorders, adverse life events, and age of onset.

Pretreatment predictors of stable remission during CAMELS included youth with higher general functioning and more positive family interactions (ie, sense of trust, open communication, and fair punishments).[72] Thus, family factors and parental relationships have a long-term impact on anxiety remission. Additionally, youth with social anxiety disorder at baseline were less likely to be in stable remission, later on, further highlighting the relationship between social anxiety disorder and poor long-term outcomes.[74] Lastly, youth with fewer traumatic and adverse life events between the original treatment and follow-up were more likely to be in stable remission. Previous studies support the relationship between stressful life events and child anxiety disorders.[75,76] Specifically, emotional neglect and psychological abuse decrease the liklihood of 4-year remission of anxiety disorders.[77] And, personality characteristics, including neuroticism, hopelessness, and external locus of control, strongly mediate the relationship between childhood maltreatment and 4-year remission.[77] These data further emphasize the importance of trauma on the long-term trajectory of anxiety disorders.

In a 16-year longitudinal study by Essau and colleagues,[78] the association between anxiety disorders with onset during two developmental periods (childhood and adolescence) was evaluated concerning long-term outcomes at age 30. Adolescent-onset anxiety disorders were associated with more negative course and outcomes than childhood-onset anxiety disorders. Specifically, adolescent-onset anxiety disorders predicted poorer total adjustment, including at work, poorer family relationships, less life satisfaction, worse coping skills, and more chronic stress in adulthood than those with childhood anxiety. Other demographic characteristics, including lower socioeconomic status, education, income, unemployment, being unmarried, or having no children, also showed unfavorable trajectories of anxiety.[79] Specifically, these characteristics contributed to a higher persistence,[80] lower probability of remission,[81] and higher risk of recurrence for anxiety.[82] Lastly, comorbid GAD and Major Depressive Disorder (MDD) are associated with a lower likelihood of remission, and this co-occurrence is associated with greater disease severity.[83,84] A summary of the predictors of recurrence and adverse long-term anxiety outcomes among youth is shown in **Table 1**.

### Predictors for Remission

Overall, predictors of remission in children and adolescents with anxiety disorders include male sex, higher socioeconomic status (SES),[85] better family functioning, lower baseline anxiety severity, absence of baseline externalizing comorbid disorders,

**Table 1**
**Predictors of recurrence of anxiety disorders in children and adolescents**

| Predictors for Recurrence | Description | Selected Reference(s) |
|---|---|---|
| Negative family interactions | • Lower sense of trust<br>• Lack of open communication | Ginsburg et al,[72] 2018 |
| Social anxiety at baseline | • Social anxiety leads to less stable remission and worse long-term outcomes | Kerns et al,[74] 2013 |
| Negative life events | • Fewer negative life events lead to a higher likelihood of stable remission | Allen et al,[75] 2008;<br>Hovens et al,[77] 2016;<br>McElroy & Hevey, 2014 |
| Adolescent-onset anxiety disorder | • Adolescent-onset leads to poorer total adjustment (work, family relationships, lower satisfaction, worse coping skills) | Essau et al,[78] 2014;<br>Beesdo et al,[11] 2010 |
| Demographic characteristics | • Lower SES and income<br>• Lower education<br>• Unemployment<br>• Being unmarried<br>• Without children | van Beljouw et al,[79] 2010;<br>Kessler et al,[80] 2012;<br>Batelaan et al,[81] 2010 |
| Comorbidity of disorders | • Co-occurring GAD and MDD lead to lower rates of remission | Kelly and Mezuk,[83] 2017;<br>Sherbourne and Wells,[84] 1997 |

and fewer negative life events (**Table 2**).[71,86,87] The most consistent predictors of remission are family functioning at baseline and being men. Youth who reported that their families had more clear rules, more trust, and higher-quality interactions at the beginning of acute treatment in the CAMS were more likely to be in remission at a 6-year follow-up.[71] Additionally, results suggest that a more significant reduction in anxiety severity and caregiver strain during CAMS predicted significantly higher levels of overall functioning in the CAMELS.[88] This highlights the fact that healthy family relationships, as well as improvements in caregiver/parental psychopathology, both play a vital role in the durability of the treatment. Specifically for social anxiety disorder, the absence of panic attacks, less avoidance, absence of comorbidity, and fewer negative life events, among others, were predictors for remission.[89] It is important to note that even if the youths do not meet diagnostic criteria for anxiety disorders, they often still experience residual symptoms,[90,91] which can negatively impact their quality of life and may increase the risk of recurrence.[92,93]

## FUTURE DIRECTIONS

It is well established that adult-type mental disorders typically emerge early in life.[94,95] Likewise, there is evidence that the course of mental illness can be modified through early intervention.[96] Yet, early intervention has been elusive for several reasons. For one, phenotypes are mostly defined lineally rather than a systems approach, which can be very complex models. So, when early identification could occur, the measurement tool's specificity and sensitivity are challenged. For example, it is now accepted that traditional service designs and allocation of resources do not align at all with the onset of the major mental disorders of adulthood, which peak during the transition from childhood to adulthood and especially in young adults,[10] making this a critical period for early intervention to alter the trajectory of mental illness.[97] Indeed, both

| Table 2 Predictors for remission of anxiety disorders in children and adolescents | | |
|---|---|---|
| **Predictors for Remission** | **Description** | **Selected Reference(s)** |
| [a]Male sex | • Males had higher rates of remission than females according to CAMELS | Ginsburg et al,[71] 2014; Asselmann and Beesdo-Baum,[87] 2015 |
| Higher SES | • Higher SES associated with higher rates of remission | Ginsburg et al,[71] 2014; Vriends et al,[85] 2007 |
| [a]Family functioning | • Clear family rules<br>• Greater trust between child and parent<br>• Higher-quality interactions | Ginsburg et al,[71] 2014; Crane et al,[88] 2021 |
| Baseline anxiety | • Lower baseline anxiety associated with greater likelihood of remission at 6-year follow-up | Ginsburg et al,[71] 2014 |
| Externalizing Disorders | • Overt and disruptive behaviors (including ODD, CD, ADHD)<br>• Absence of comorbidity associated with higher rates of remission | Ginsburg et al,[71] 2014 |
| Negative Life Events | • Fewer negative life events associated with higher remission rates | Ginsburg et al,[71] 2014; Allen et al., 2008; Asselmann and Beesdo-Baum,[87] 2015; Essau et al,[86] 2002 |
| Caregiver Strain | • Reduction in caregiver strain during CAMS predicted higher levels of overall functioning in CAMELS | Crane et al,[88] 2021 |
| Social Anxiety Disorder | • Absence of panic attacks<br>• Less avoidance<br>• Lack of comorbid psychiatric disorders | Vriends et al,[89] 2014 |

[a] Most consistent predictors of remission were family functioning at baseline and male sex.

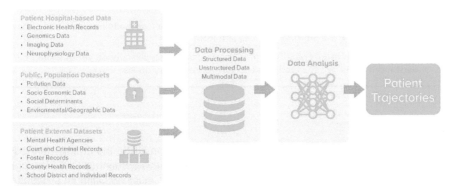

**Fig. 3.** Data processing model and artificial intelligence-based data analysis for neuropsychiatric patient trajectories. Through collaboration with CCHMC and Oak Ridge National Laboratory.

universal and targeted prevention programs hold promise for altering trajectories leading to psychiatric disorders, although it is essential that these are guided by a deep understanding of the developmental epidemiology and etiology of anxiety disorders.[98]

More recently, technological and analytic advances have created opportunities for empirically-driven early identification of psychiatric disorders.[99] High-performance computing has been used to place complex models of emergence of psychiatric disorders into a high-dimensional space and compute the possible combinations that represent the phenotype (**Fig. 3**). This approach enables very fast (exaflop) computations of large quantities of clinical data to drive early identification of unfolding disorders. These computational and systems advances have the potential to guide clinicians, in real-time, to identify anxiety disorders earlier.

## SUMMARY

Anxiety disorders are early-emerging and frequently are accompanied by significant functional impairment and accumulated disability for children later in life. These disorders often show a persistent trajectory beginning in childhood, with both homotypic and heterotypic courses. The onset of anxiety disorder development in children can predict the subsequent persistence of symptoms later in life and specific anxiety disorders have varied longitudinal trends. Of note, the COVID-19 pandemic has dramatically increased anxiety symptom prevalence among children and adolescents and highlights a need for intervention and treatment among this group. The combination of male sex, higher socioeconomic status, and fewer negative life events have been shown to predict improved remission rates, among other factors. More work is needed to identify specific risk factors and understand the complex underlying biopsychosocial mechanisms and interactions for the development of disease to improve outcomes and address rising anxiety rates in youth.

## CLINICS CARE POINTS

- Clinicians should understand the general longitudinal trajectories of pediatric anxiety disorders so they can intervene early and prevent subsequent development of later or worsening disease
- Understanding the age of onset of specific disorders as well as sex-specific trends among anxiety prevalence allow providers to better anticipate and identify the development of specific disorders among this age group
- The rising prevalence of anxiety disorders among children and adolescents during the COVID-19 pandemic is a pressing public health issue
- Predictors for both recurrence and remission of anxiety disorders among youth should be understood by clinicians to identify risk factors for refractory disease

## ACKNOWLEDGMENTS

This work was supported by the Yung Family Foundation (JRS), the Eunice Kennedy Shriver National Institute of Child Health and Human Development (NICHD) through R01HD099775 (JRS) and R01HD098757 (JRS), and by Cincinnati Children's Hospital Medical Center, United States under Strategic Partnership Projects agreement NFE-21-08617. This book article has been partially authored by UT-Battelle, LLC under Contract No. DE-AC05-00OR22725 with the US Department of Energy.

## DISCLOSURES

Dr J.R. Strawn has received research support from the Yung Family Foundation, the National Institutes of Health (NIMH/NIEHS/NICHD), the National Center for Advancing Translational Sciences, United States, the Patient-Centered Outcomes Research Institute, United States and Abbvie, United States. He has received material support from Myriad Health and royalties from three texts (Springer). Dr J.R. Strawn serves as an author for *UpToDate* and an Associate Editor for *Current Psychiatry* and has provided consultation to the FDA, Cereval, and IntraCellular Therapeutics. Views expressed within this article represent those of the authors and are not intended to represent the position of NIMH, United States, the National Institutes of Health, United States, or the Department of Health and Human Services.

## REFERENCES

1. Force USPST, Mangione CM, Barry MJ, et al. Screening for anxiety in children and adolescents: us preventive services task force recommendation statement. JAMA 2022;328(14):1438–44.
2. Viswanathan M, Wallace IF, Cook Middleton J, et al. Screening for anxiety in children and adolescents: evidence report and systematic review for the US preventive services task force. JAMA 2022;328(14):1445–55.
3. Walkup JT, Green CM, Strawn JR. Screening for pediatric anxiety disorders. JAMA 2022;328(14):1399–401.
4. Penninx BW, Pine DS, Holmes EA, et al. Anxiety disorders. Lancet 2021; 397(10277):914–27.
5. Finsaas MC, Bufferd SJ, Dougherty LR, et al. Preschool psychiatric disorders: homotypic and heterotypic continuity through middle childhood and early adolescence. Psychol Med 2018;48(13):2159–68.
6. Merikangas KR, He JP, Brody D, et al. Prevalence and treatment of mental disorders among US children in the 2001-2004 NHANES. Pediatrics 2010;125(1):75–81.
7. Fichter MM, Quadflieg N, Fischer UC, et al. Twenty-five-year course and outcome in anxiety and depression in the upper bavarian longitudinal community study. Acta Psychiatr Scand 2010;122(1):75–85.
8. Steinsbekk S, Ranum B, Wichstrom L. Prevalence and course of anxiety disorders and symptoms from preschool to adolescence: a 6-wave community study. J Child Psychol Psychiatry 2022;63(5):527–34.
9. Becker ES, Rinck M, Turke V, et al. Epidemiology of specific phobia subtypes: findings from the dresden mental health study. Eur Psychiatry 2007;22(2):69–74.
10. Kessler RC, Berglund P, Demler O, et al. Lifetime prevalence and age-of-onset distributions of DSM-IV disorders in the national comorbidity survey replication. Arch Gen Psychiatry 2005;62(6):593–602.
11. Beesdo K, Pine DS, Lieb R, et al. Incidence and risk patterns of anxiety and depressive disorders and categorization of generalized anxiety disorder. Arch Gen Psychiatry 2010;67(1):47–57.
12. Strawn JR, Lu L, Peris TS, et al. Research review: pediatric anxiety disorders - what have we learnt in the last 10 years? J Child Psychol Psychiatry 2021;62(2):114–39.
13. Beesdo-Baum K, Knappe S, Asselmann E, et al. The 'Early Developmental Stages of Psychopathology (EDSP) study': a 20-year review of methods and findings. Soc Psychiatry Psychiatr Epidemiol 2015;50(6):851–66.

14. Beesdo-Baum K, Knappe S. Developmental epidemiology of anxiety disorders. Child Adolesc Psychiatr Clin N Am 2012;21(3):457–78.
15. Arthur M. Institute for health metrics and evaluation. Nurs Stand 2014;28(42):32.
16. Beesdo K, Knappe S, Pine DS. Anxiety and anxiety disorders in children and adolescents: developmental issues and implications for DSM-V. Psychiatr Clin North Am 2009;32(3):483–524.
17. Merikangas KR, He JP, Burstein M, et al. Lifetime prevalence of mental disorders in U.S. Adolescents: results from the national comorbidity survey replication–adolescent supplement (NCS-A). J Am Acad Child Adolesc Psychiatry 2010; 49(10):980–9.
18. Racine N, McArthur BA, Cooke JE, et al. Global Prevalence of depressive and anxiety symptoms in children and adolescents during COVID-19: a meta-analysis. JAMA Pediatr 2021;175(11):1142–50.
19. Copeland WE, Angold A, Shanahan L, et al. Longitudinal patterns of anxiety from childhood to adulthood: the Great Smoky mountains study. J Am Acad Child Adolesc Psychiatry 2014;53(1):21–33.
20. Spence SH, Zubrick SR, Lawrence D. A profile of social, separation and generalized anxiety disorders in an Australian nationally representative sample of children and adolescents: prevalence, comorbidity and correlates. Aust N Z J Psychiatry 2018;52(5):446–60.
21. Bandelow B, Michaelis S. Epidemiology of anxiety disorders in the 21st century. Dialogues Clin Neurosci 2015;17(3):327–35.
22. Somers JM, Goldner EM, Waraich P, et al. Prevalence and incidence studies of anxiety disorders: a systematic review of the literature. Can J Psychiatry 2006; 51(2):100–13.
23. Lijster JM, Dierckx B, Utens EM, et al. The age of onset of anxiety disorders. Can J Psychiatry 2017;62(4):237–46.
24. Tiirikainen K, Haravuori H, Ranta K, et al. Psychometric properties of the 7-item Generalized Anxiety Disorder Scale (GAD-7) in a large representative sample of Finnish adolescents. Psychiatry Res 2019;272:30–5.
25. Duan L, Shao X, Wang Y, et al. An investigation of mental health status of children and adolescents in China during the outbreak of COVID-19. J Affect Disord 2020;275:112–8.
26. Zhao J, Xing X, Wang M. Psychometric properties of the spence Children's anxiety scale (SCAS) in mainland Chinese children and adolescents. J Anxiety Disord 2012;26(7):728–36.
27. Tang S, Xiang M, Cheung T, et al. Mental health and its correlates among children and adolescents during COVID-19 school closure: the importance of parent-child discussion. J Affect Disord 2021;279:353–60.
28. Warner EN, Strawn JR. Risk factors of pediatric anxiety disorders. Psychiatr Clin: Updates in Anxiety Treatment 2022;33:1.
29. Yap MB, Pilkington PD, Ryan SM, et al. Parental factors associated with depression and anxiety in young people: a systematic review and meta-analysis. J Affect Disord 2014;156:8–23.
30. Osmanagaoglu N, Creswell C, Dodd HF. Intolerance of Uncertainty, anxiety, and worry in children and adolescents: a meta-analysis. J Affect Disord 2018;225: 80–90.
31. Strawn J.R., Mills J.A., Schroeder H.K., et al., The Impact of COVID-19 Infection and Characterization of "Long COVID" in Adolescents With Anxiety Disorders: A Prospective Longitudinal Study, J Am Acad Child Adolesc Psychiatry.

2023:S0890-8567(23)00065-5. https://doi.org/10.1016/j.jaac.2022.12.027. (in press).

32. Lowe B, Decker O, Muller S, et al. Validation and standardization of the generalized anxiety disorder screener (GAD-7) in the general population. Med Care 2008;46(3):266–74.

33. Wehry AM, Beesdo-Baum K, Hennelly MM, et al. Assessment and treatment of anxiety disorders in children and adolescents. Curr Psychiatry Rep 2015; 17(7):52.

34. Kim-Cohen J, Caspi A, Moffitt TE, et al. Prior juvenile diagnoses in adults with mental disorder: developmental follow-back of a prospective-longitudinal cohort. Arch Gen Psychiatry 2003;60(7):709–17.

35. Cohen JR, Andrews AR, Davis MM, et al. Anxiety and depression during childhood and adolescence: testing theoretical models of continuity and discontinuity. J Abnorm Child Psychol 2018;46(6):1295–308.

36. Ferdinand RF, Dieleman G, Ormel J, et al. Homotypic versus heterotypic continuity of anxiety symptoms in young adolescents: evidence for distinctions between DSM-IV subtypes. J Abnorm Child Psychol 2007;35(3):325–33.

37. Wittchen HU, Kessler RC, Pfister H, et al. Why do people with anxiety disorders become depressed? A prospective-longitudinal community study. Acta Psychiatr Scand Suppl 2000;(406):14–23.

38. Copeland WE, Shanahan L, Costello EJ, et al. Childhood and adolescent psychiatric disorders as predictors of young adult disorders. Arch Gen Psychiatry 2009;66(7):764–72.

39. Betts KS, Baker P, Alati R, et al. The natural history of internalizing behaviours from adolescence to emerging adulthood: findings from the Australian Temperament Project. Psychol Med 2016;46(13):2815–27.

40. Foley DL, Goldston DB, Costello EJ, et al. Proximal psychiatric risk factors for suicidality in youth: the Great Smoky Mountains Study. Arch Gen Psychiatry 2006;63(9):1017–24.

41. Husky MM, Olfson M, He JP, et al. Twelve-month suicidal symptoms and use of services among adolescents: results from the National Comorbidity Survey. Psychiatr Serv 2012;63(10):989–96.

42. Ahlen J, Ghaderi A. Dimension-specific symptom patterns in trajectories of broad anxiety: a longitudinal prospective study in school-aged children. Dev Psychopathol 2020;32(1):31–41.

43. Weems CF. Developmental trajectories of childhood anxiety: identifying continuity and change in anxious emotion. Dev Rev 2008;28:488–502. https://doi.org/10.1016/j.dr.2008.01.00.

44. Pattwell SS, Lee FS, Casey BJ. Fear learning and memory across adolescent development: hormones and behavior special issue: puberty and adolescence. Horm Behav 2013;64(2):380–9.

45. Pattwell SS, Liston C, Jing D, et al. Dynamic changes in neural circuitry during adolescence are associated with persistent attenuation of fear memories. Nat Commun 2016;7:11475.

46. Shear K, Jin R, Ruscio AM, et al. Prevalence and correlates of estimated DSM-IV child and adult separation anxiety disorder in the National Comorbidity Survey Replication. Am J Psychiatry 2006;163(6):1074–83.

47. Foley D, Rutter M, Pickles A, et al. Informant disagreement for separation anxiety disorder. J Am Acad Child Adolesc Psychiatry 2004;43(4):452–60.

48. Kossowsky J, Pfaltz MC, Schneider S, et al. The separation anxiety hypothesis of panic disorder revisited: a meta-analysis. Am J Psychiatry 2013;170(7): 768–81.

49. Simonoff E, Pickles A, Meyer JM, et al. The Virginia Twin Study of Adolescent Behavioral Development. Influences of age, sex, and impairment on rates of disorder. Arch Gen Psychiatry 1997;54(9):801–8.

50. Lavallee K, Herren C, Blatter-Meunier J, Adornetto C, In-Albon T, Schneider S. Early predictors of separation anxiety disorder: early stranger anxiety, parental pathology and prenatal factors. Psychopathology 2011;44(6):354–61.

51. Newman MG, Shin KE, Zuellig AR. Developmental risk factors in generalized anxiety disorder and panic disorder. J Affect Disord 2016;206:94–102.

52. Social anxiety disorder: recognition, assessment and treatment. Guidelines: National Institute for Health and Care Excellence; 2013.

53. Beesdo K, Bittner A, Pine DS, et al. Incidence of social anxiety disorder and the consistent risk for secondary depression in the first three decades of life. Arch Gen Psychiatry 2007;64(8):903–12.

54. Black JJ, Clark DB, Martin CS, et al. Course of alcohol symptoms and social anxiety disorder from adolescence to young adulthood. Alcohol Clin Exp Res 2015;39(6):1008–15.

55. Buckner JD, Schmidt NB, Lang AR, et al. Specificity of social anxiety disorder as a risk factor for alcohol and cannabis dependence. J Psychiatr Res 2008;42(3): 230–9.

56. Ranoyen I, Lydersen S, Larose TL, et al. Developmental course of anxiety and depression from adolescence to young adulthood in a prospective Norwegian clinical cohort. Eur Child Adolesc Psychiatry 2018;27(11):1413–23.

57. Crone EA, Dahl RE. Understanding adolescence as a period of social-affective engagement and goal flexibility. Nat Rev Neurosci 2012;13(9):636–50.

58. Showraki M, Showraki T, Brown K. Generalized anxiety disorder: revisited. Psychiatr Q 2020;91(3):905–14.

59. Costello EJ, Mustillo S, Erkanli A, et al. Prevalence and development of psychiatric disorders in childhood and adolescence. Arch Gen Psychiatry 2003;60(8): 837–44.

60. Dobson ET, Croarkin PE, Schroeder HK, et al. Bridging anxiety and depression: a network approach in anxious adolescents. J Affect Disord 2021;280(Pt A): 305–14.

61. Kessler RC, Gruber M, Hettema JM, et al. Co-morbid major depression and generalized anxiety disorders in the National Comorbidity Survey follow-up. Psychol Med 2008;38(3):365–74.

62. Nelemans SA, Hale WW, Branje SJT, et al. Individual differences in anxiety trajectories from Grades 2 to 8: impact of the middle school transition. Dev Psychopathol 2018;30(4):1487–501.

63. Swan AJ, Kendall PC, Olino T, et al. Results from the child/adolescent anxiety multimodal longitudinal study (CAMELS): functional outcomes. J Consult Clin Psychol 2018;86(9):738–50.

64. Gao W, Ping S, Liu X. Gender differences in depression, anxiety, and stress among college students: a longitudinal study from China. J Affect Disord 2020;263:292–300.

65. Al-Qaisy LM. The relation of depression and anxiety in academic achievement among group of university students. Int J Psychol Couns 2011;3(5):96–100.

66. Wong JG, Cheung EP, Chan KK, et al. Web-based survey of depression, anxiety and stress in first-year tertiary education students in Hong Kong. Aust N Z J Psychiatry 2006;40(9):777–82.
67. Crocetti E, Klimstra T, Keijsers L, et al. Anxiety trajectories and identity development in adolescence: a five-wave longitudinal study. J Youth Adolesc 2009; 38(6):839–49.
68. Legerstee JS, Verhulst FC, Robbers SC, et al. Gender-specific developmental trajectories of anxiety during adolescence: determinants and outcomes. The TRAILS study. J Can Acad Child Adolesc Psychiatry 2013;22(1):26–34.
69. Barrett PM, Farrell LJ, Ollendick TH, et al. Long-term outcomes of an Australian universal prevention trial of anxiety and depression symptoms in children and youth: an evaluation of the friends program. J Clin Child Adolesc Psychol 2006;35(3):403–11.
70. Bushnell GA, Talati A, Wickramaratne PJ, et al. Trajectories of childhood anxiety disorders in two generations at high risk. Depress Anxiety 2020;37(6):521–31.
71. Ginsburg GS, Becker EM, Keeton CP, et al. Naturalistic follow-up of youths treated for pediatric anxiety disorders. JAMA Psychiatr 2014;71(3):310–8.
72. Ginsburg GS, Becker-Haimes EM, Keeton C, et al. Results from the child/adolescent anxiety multimodal extended long-term study (CAMELS): primary anxiety outcomes. J Am Acad Child Adolesc Psychiatry 2018;57(7):471–80.
73. Walkup JT, Albano AM, Piacentini J, et al. Cognitive behavioral therapy, sertraline, or a combination in childhood anxiety. N Engl J Med 2008;359(26): 2753–66.
74. Kerns CM, Read KL, Klugman J, et al. Cognitive behavioral therapy for youth with social anxiety: differential short and long-term treatment outcomes. J Anxiety Disord 2013;27(2):210–5.
75. Allen JL, Rapee RM, Sandberg S. Severe life events and chronic adversities as antecedents to anxiety in children: a matched control study. J Abnorm Child Psychol 2008;36(7):1047–56.
76. Mc Elroy S, Hevey D. Relationship between adverse early experiences, stressors, psychosocial resources and wellbeing. Child Abuse Negl 2014; 38(1):65–75. https://doi.org/10.1016/j.chiabu.2013.07.017.
77. Hovens JG, Giltay EJ, van Hemert AM, et al. Childhood maltreatment and the course of depressive and anxiety disorders: the contribution of personality characteristics. Depress Anxiety 2016;33(1):27–34.
78. Essau CA, Lewinsohn PM, Olaya B, et al. Anxiety disorders in adolescents and psychosocial outcomes at age 30. J Affect Disord 2014;163:125–32.
79. van Beljouw IM, Verhaak PF, Cuijpers P, et al. The course of untreated anxiety and depression, and determinants of poor one-year outcome: a one-year cohort study. BMC Psychiatry 2010;10:86.
80. Kessler RC, Petukhova M, Sampson NA, et al. Twelve-month and lifetime prevalence and lifetime morbid risk of anxiety and mood disorders in the United States. Int J Methods Psychiatr Res 2012;21(3):169–84.
81. Batelaan NM, de Graaf R, Penninx BW, et al. The 2-year prognosis of panic episodes in the general population. Psychol Med 2010;40(1):147–57.
82. Scholten WD, Batelaan NM, van Balkom AJ, et al. Recurrence of anxiety disorders and its predictors. J Affect Disord 2013;147(1–3):180–5.
83. Kelly KM, Mezuk B. Predictors of remission from generalized anxiety disorder and major depressive disorder. J Affect Disord 2017;208:467–74.
84. Sherbourne CD, Wells KB. Course of depression in patients with comorbid anxiety disorders. J Affect Disord 1997;43(3):245–50.

85. Vriends N, Becker ES, Meyer A, et al. Recovery from social phobia in the community and its predictors: data from a longitudinal epidemiological study. J Anxiety Disord 2007;21(3):320–37.
86. Essau CA, Conradt J, Petermann F. Course and outcome of anxiety disorders in adolescents. J Anxiety Disord 2002;16(1):67–81.
87. Asselmann E, Beesdo-Baum K. Predictors of the course of anxiety disorders in adolescents and young adults. Curr Psychiatry Rep 2015;17(2):7.
88. Crane ME, Norris LA, Frank HE, et al. Impact of treatment improvement on long-term anxiety: results from CAMS and CAMELS. J Consult Clin Psychol 2021; 89(2):126–33.
89. Vriends N, Bolt OC, Kunz SM. Social anxiety disorder, a lifelong disorder? A review of the spontaneous remission and its predictors. Acta Psychiatr Scand 2014;130(2):109–22.
90. Zimmerman M, Martinez J, Attiullah N, et al. Why do some depressed outpatients who are not in remission according to the Hamilton depression rating scale nonetheless consider themselves to be in remission? Depress Anxiety 2012;29(10):891–5.
91. Rodriguez BF, Weisberg RB, Pagano ME, et al. Characteristics and predictors of full and partial recovery from generalized anxiety disorder in primary care patients. J Nerv Ment Dis 2006;194(2):91–7.
92. Paykel ES. Partial remission, residual symptoms, and relapse in depression. Dialogues Clin Neurosci 2008;10(4):431–7.
93. Judd LL, Akiskal HS, Maser JD, et al. Major depressive disorder: a prospective study of residual subthreshold depressive symptoms as predictor of rapid relapse. J Affect Disord 1998;50(2–3):97–108.
94. Burcusa SL, Iacono WG. Risk for recurrence in depression. Clin Psychol Rev 2007;27(8):959–85.
95. Gibb SJ, Fergusson DM, Horwood LJ. Burden of psychiatric disorder in young adulthood and life outcomes at age 30. Br J Psychiatry 2010;197(2):122–7.
96. Correll CU, Galling B, Pawar A, et al. Comparison of early intervention services vs treatment as usual for early-phase psychosis: a systematic review, meta-analysis, and meta-regression. JAMA Psychiatr 2018;75(6):555–65.
97. McGorry PD, Mei C. Early intervention in youth mental health: progress and future directions. Evid Based Ment Health 2018;21(4):182–4.
98. Teubert D, Pinquart M. A meta-analytic review on the prevention of symptoms of anxiety in children and adolescents. J Anxiety Disord 2011;25:1046–59.
99. Pestian J, Santel D, Sorter M, et al. A machine learning approach to identifying changes in suicidal language. Suicide Life Threat Behav 2020;50(5):939–47.
100. Dalsgaard S, Thorsteinsson E, Trabjerg BB, et al. Incidence rates and cumulative incidences of the full spectrum of diagnosed mental disorders in childhood and adolescence. JAMA Psychiatr 2020;77(2):155–64.

# The Impact of COVID-19 on Anxiety Disorders in Youth
## Coping with Stress, Worry, and Recovering from a Pandemic

Lisa R. Fortuna, MD, MPH[a],*, Isabella C. Brown, MA[b],
Gesean G. Lewis Woods, MA[b], Michelle V. Porche, EdD[c]

## KEYWORDS

- Anxiety disorders • COVID-19 pandemic • Special populations • Disabilities
- Children • Adolescents • System of care • Schools

## KEY POINTS

- The COVID-19 pandemic has had a disproportionate impact on communities of color and on under-resourced communities by imposing additional psychosocial stressors that contributed to persistent anxiety, worries, and distress for many children and adolescents.
- Anxiety disorders and stress have been notable aspects of young people's experience during the pandemic, and it will be important to consider ways to respond to anxiety and stress as we move into a recovery phase.
- Intersectional identities are relevant to the experiences of young people during the pandemic, and this is important to think about for planning prevention and treatment interventions for anxiety and related stressors.
- Youth from minoritized backgrounds with mental health and learning disabilities that predated the pandemic are potentially more vulnerable to experiencing anxiety disorders.
- A combined clinical and system of care approach that includes identifying and addressing the specific needs of children and adolescents, implementing prevention, and resilience-promoting interventions within clinical services, schools, families, and the community are needed going forward.

[a] Department of Psychiatry and Behavioral Sciences, University of California, San Francisco, Zuckerberg San Francisco General Hospital, 1001 Potrero, Avenue, Building 5 Room 7M8, San Francisco, CA 94110, USA; [b] Berkeley School of Education, University of California, Berkeley, 2121 Berkeley Way, 4th Floor, Berkeley, CA 94720-1670, USA; [c] Department of Psychiatry and Behavioral Sciences, University of California, San Francisco, 1001 Potrero Avenue, Building 5 Room 7M2, San Francisco, CA 94110, USA
* Corresponding author.
E-mail address: lisa.fortuna@ucsf.edu

Child Adolesc Psychiatric Clin N Am 32 (2023) 531–542
https://doi.org/10.1016/j.chc.2023.02.002
1056-4993/23/© 2023 Elsevier Inc. All rights reserved.
childpsych.theclinics.com

## INTRODUCTION

The COVID-19 pandemic has resulted in a dramatic increase in the rate of anxiety problems and social risks among children, adolescents, and young adults in the United States and globally. The stressors heralded in by the pandemic disproportionately affected racial- minoritized and ethnic-minoritized school-age children, adolescents, and young adults.[1] This is in context of pre-existing social inequities and growing mental health services needs experienced by children and adolescents more broadly. Even before the pandemic, there were already escalating rates of inpatient visits for suicide, suicidal ideation, and self-injury for children aged 1 to 17 years old, and just in the first 10 months of 2020, there was a 151% increase in these concerns for children aged 10 to 14.[2] There has been a 61% increase in the rate of self-reported mental health needs since 2005.[3] Anxiety has been an important problem to consider since the pandemic; one national survey found that more than one in four children report sleep problems due to worries, feeling unhappy, and anxious.[4] In this review, we offer findings from recent studies on anxiety, particularly patterns identified during the pandemic. We also consider case illustrations and recommendations for assessment, clinical care, and system-based approaches for treatment and prevention.

### Pandemic-Driven Anxiety and Mental Health Problems in Children and Adolescents

The mental health needs of youth shifted during the COVID-19 pandemic. Rates of psychological distress among young people, including symptoms of anxiety disorders (eg, generalized anxiety disorder, social anxiety disorders, separation anxiety) and other broad anxiety symptoms (eg, worry and fears), and depression have worsened. Recent research covering 80,000 youths globally found that depressive and anxiety symptoms doubled during the pandemic with 20% of youth reporting that they are experiencing significant anxiety symptoms.[5] There are several potential reasons. During the pandemic, children, adolescents, and young adults have faced unprecedented challenges as the pandemic radically changed their world, including how children and youths have attended school and been socialized. They missed important events, time with friends and teachers, and time with relatives. A recent study[6] showed that children who already had subjective anxiety about their parents and themselves at baseline also had increased anxiety sensitivity, including what has been termed coronavirus anxiety (eg, feeling dizzy, lightheaded, faint, paralyzed, frozen, or other intense anxiety feelings when thinking about or exposed to information about the coronavirus). A study of distal and proximal predictors of child mental health found the pandemic to be a mediator between maternal history of adverse childhood experiences and her child's traumatic stress symptoms, which were also associated with internalizing symptoms before the pandemic.[7] Loneliness, social distancing, and internet usage also strongly correlated with mental health-related issues including stress, anxiety, and depression.[6]

   Youths with intersectional identities, such as minoritized youths with low socioeconomic status, homeless youths, and lesbian, gay, bisexual, transgender and queer (LGBTQ) youths, have been especially vulnerable during the pandemic given the increased risks they have faced. LGBTQ youths have experienced disproportionate negative outcomes in housing stability, employment, and mental health and trauma due to COVID-19 resulting from the combination of their sexual and gender identity discrimination, foster care involvement, and lower socioeconomic status.[8] Youths from the Asian and Pacific Islander communities have experienced an increase in abuse and discrimination, given the uptick in anti-Asian rhetoric and hate crimes that escalated during the pandemic.[9] These discriminatory experiences have continued unabated and have resulted in the clinical presentation of generalized anxiety, social anxiety, and depression for many children and adolescents who, as a result, worry about their safety and that of their elders.[10]

Children, youths, and their families experienced multiple stressors throughout the pandemic. Some may have lost access to mental health care, social services, income, food, or housing. Some children may have had COVID-19 themselves, suffered from long COVID symptoms, or lost a loved one to COVID-related illness. Recent published estimates suggest that more than 200,000 children in the United States have lost a parent or grandparent caregiver to COVID-19.[11] COVID-19 disproportionately affected the Black, Latinx, and other children and adolescents of color, where adult family members were more likely to be affected front-line workers. Cumulative data from the state of California indicate that the Latinos overall, and Latino children specifically, are over-represented in both infection rates and mortality rates.[12] A study found that presenting to a health clinic with possible COVID-19 symptoms, being polymerase chain reaction (PCR)-positive for COVID-19, or being hospitalized with a verified disease, posed a significant risk to children and adolescents and the development of psychological disorders, including anxiety, depression, posttraumatic stress disorder, and sleep disturbances.[13]

Spencer and collegues[14] assessed mental health symptoms and social risks during COVID-19 versus before the pandemic among urban, racial- minority and ethnic-minority school-aged children. The analysis included caregivers of 168 children (aged 5 to 11 years old) recruited from an urban safety-net hospital-based pediatric primary care practice with follow-up from September 2019 to January 2021.[14] The researchers found that children had significantly higher levels of emotional and behavioral symptoms mid-pandemic versus pre-pandemic across all domains. During the pandemic, significantly more children reported clinical concerns and had positive pediatric symptom checklist screenings in primary care and mental health services. The caregivers reported significantly more social risks and behavioral changes in their children during the pandemic. The researchers found significant associations between less school assignment completion, increased screen time, and caregiver depression with worse mid-pandemic mental health in children. Although other research has suggested that bullying, cyberbullying, sexting, and fighting showed only small or no increases, anxiety and depression have dramatically increased relative to before the pandemic.[15]

One study pooled the estimates obtained from the first year of the COVID-19 pandemic[5] that suggested one in five youth were experiencing clinically elevated anxiety symptoms. The authors concluded that an influx of mental health care utilization is expected, and the allocation of resources to address child and adolescent mental health concerns is essential. There was a correlation observed between mental health symptoms during the pandemic and the number of social risks before the pandemic. Girls and LGBTQ youths were particularly vulnerable during the months following the shelter-in-place requirements that were initiated in March 2020. Girls and LGBTQ youths experienced a greater risk of anxiety and depression, even as cyberbullying and other online threats were relatively unchanged. This increase in symptoms was at least in part attributed to a reduction in access to social support and an increase in psychosocial stressors in the context of the pandemic.[15] Unhoused youths were at particular risk. One study found that young adults experiencing homelessness experienced more stressors compared with housed peers, described unmet basic needs, frustration, and anxiety, and increases in risk behaviors including substance use.[16] Youths with chronic medical conditions such as diabetes were also at risk of poor disease management, stress, and anxiety which increased their vulnerability to medical emergencies during the pandemic.[17]

A recent systematic review and meta-analysis examined the prevalence of anxiety disorders in the general population during the COVID-19 pandemic. Delpino et al. (2022) reviewed 194 studies that assessed the prevalence of anxiety among the general population globally during the pandemic. The general prevalence of anxiety was 35.1%, affecting approximately 851,000 participants across the studies. The prevalence in low- income and middle-income countries (35.1%; 95% CI: 29.5%–41.0%) was similar compared to high-income countries (34.7%; 95% CI: 29.6%–40.1%).[18] In addition to reporting on the prevalence of anxiety disorders and the high impact across demographics, the authors note that one in 10 cases with anxiety during COVID-19 may be continuing to live with clinically meaningful anxiety symptoms. The challenge is identifying and helping the children and youths who are most in need.

## CHILDREN WITH SPECIAL NEEDS: RETURNING TO SCHOOL AND CATCHING UP

Crucially, remote learning at the height of the pandemic disrupted educational trajectories and school-based services. Children requiring special education and other specialized services struggled more than peers without such needs.[19] It is important to consider how the combination of educationally-based stressors, learning disabilities, and other social factors can contribute to anxiety and exacerbate other preexisting developmental and mental health conditions. The following clinical case studies illustrate some of these factors.

### Clinical Case Studies

#### Carl's story

*"Carl" is a 14-year-old boy with inattentive Attention Deficit Hyperactivity Disorder (ADHD) and dyslexia. Right before the pandemic, he had started his freshman year at a new school with all new peers. He was taking prescribed ADHD medication, but not enough to help him fully manage his restlessness in the classroom. He faced additional pressures across racial differences as one of the few Black students at the school, too often subjected to disproportional discipline, as was the case for other students of color at the high school. He started to complain that he hated school because of these interactions and he did not have enough positive experiences to strike a balance. He said that his classes were too difficult and that it was too hard to stay on task. School was especially challenging when all instruction was conducted via Zoom during shelter-in-place. His parents struggled with how to best support him–taking care of his emotional needs or responding to pressure from teachers to increase their surveillance to keep him on task. They felt there was no middle ground.*

*For Carl, even physical education was hard when he was sheltering at home because he felt self-conscious exercising in front of his family in the only available space of the living room. He experienced feelings of anxiety and tension because he was unable to read content on the web pages for assignments. Now back at school, he is distracted and does not want to show up for class anymore. His struggles are complicated by his ADHD and learning disabilities. The teachers in his classes require that he do what others are doing, and he feels pressure to read as quickly as his peers in his Language Arts class. He cannot keep up but does not want to show it.*

*To make the classes more interesting, the teachers use "popcorn" pedagogy, where students randomly select the next person to talk or to read after they have finished their turn. This strategy is engaging for neurotypical students but can make students with learning differences anxious, invoking a fight or flight response. When this happens, Carl often wants to crawl under the table, but instead asks repeatedly to go to the bathroom to get out of class.*

*During COVID-19 remote learning, students with disabilities like Carl lacked the one-on-one classroom paraprofessional aid they had previously, and schools continue to be short-staffed in providing this resource. At home, at least Carl was able to get up and walk around more easily, using this as an escape strategy when stressed. However, with access to the entire internet to escape, Carl was doing many online activities outside of the class curriculum. Although this helped him manage his anxiety, he ultimately fell further behind. Now he has further to catch up.*

### Clinical Considerations

One study[19] suggested that telehealth and remote learning were often complicated for children with disabilities, widening related disparities as youths re-enter school. Clinical and educational services were not reliably available in school settings. Families are understandably frustrated if their child has been unable to access services legally mandated through the child's Individualized Educational Plan (IEP). An important first step is to reassess a child's special education and emotional needs, implement an IEP that is responsive to the child's current needs, and, whenever possible, in coordination with the mental health clinician. Some considerations.

- Medication checks are an opportunity to ask about other issues, such as isolation and loneliness, frustration, and stress, which medications cannot help. For youth with increasing inattention and/or hyperactivity, the clinical impulse may be to increase ADHD medications or add on an antidepressant or anxiolytic medication for anxiety. In clinical situations such as Carl's, it is important to examine the full range of circumstances influencing symptoms; assessing what educational, social, and behavioral supports are needed is an essential first step.
- Find out about environmental issues. Intrusive thoughts may be directly connected to pandemic-related worries and hard for the child to stop when the child is stressed and lonely or worried about persistent stressors at home.
- Provide children with strategies to manage their negative self-talk like "this is hard and yet I have to do this all again tomorrow" and address overwhelming thoughts about coping and readjusting to the school setting.
- Offer school-based behavioral health services that include evidence-based treatments such as cognitive behavioral therapy and emotional regulation strategies.

### Linda's Story

*Linda is a 5th-grade Latina girl with immigrant parents who are bilingual but Spanish-dominant. Linda is diagnosed with autism spectrum disorder (ASD) but has received limited services. Her ASD symptoms are mild and she is in mainstream classrooms and had just begun receiving special education support before the pandemic started. Her parents are supportive but unsure how to help her and have received little useful information about ASD. Linda's sensory issues made remote learning challenging for a variety of reasons. For example, when Linda's computer was on the Zoom gallery view, there was too much going on, especially when many were learning how to use technology. There were often multiple students unmuted at the same time, and the transmitted background noise from their homes was stressful.*

*The Zoom video was visually overstimulating for Linda. Her neurotypical peers were able to filter out these distractions, but Linda could not and she became increasingly anxious. She sometimes responded to this overstimulation by skimming, for example, tapping and engaging in repetitive movements that were soothing to her, but these behaviors seemed disruptive for other students, and the teacher and staff responded negatively. Before the pandemic, Linda might also respond to overstimulation by eloping–running away, leaving the classroom, wandering away–which the staff could respond to by gently guiding her back to her seat. However, on Zoom, it was a struggle to keep her engaged in front of the computer as her anxiety rose. The teachers required that she keep her camera on for accountability and that she must remain in her seat; now back at school, the same expectations apply.*

*Like other children with ASD, Linda's senses can go into overdrive, and as a result, her anxiety can escalate. This is usually related to sounds, and every noise feels that much louder for her than for her peers. When computer sounds or classroom noise feel too loud, her head feels like it is on a swivel, so she sometimes hits her head "to put it back together." This behavior draws the attention of her classmates, resulting in increased anxiety for Linda.*

### Clinical considerations

Students like Linda had difficulty using virtual platforms for education and could not take the breaks they needed. School schedules were not typical schedules and often not a full day of classes. So, the teachers may have felt that they could go without breaks because of these fewer hours. These assumptions may not have been congruent with the needs of students in special education. Now back at school and in the classroom, the youths may be experiencing a need to catch up from losses in their educational, social, and developmental progress. The peers may misunderstand self-soothing behaviors. They then might tease or bully the student, who might then become dysregulated or withdrawn.

Clinicians and teachers should not assume that students with ASD are uninterested in being around children their age. Withdrawal may be a response to poor experiences with peers. Avoidance behaviors may have been exacerbated by the transition to virtual learning and then back to in-person learning, as transitions are a known challenge for those with ASD. Actions that can help include:

- During virtual learning, asking questions about isolation and loneliness. Upon return to in-person instruction, asking about other activities, friends, hobbies, or sports that can help engage the child and getting information about this from parents as well as from teachers.
- Knowing more about the child's academic strengths and areas of need helps to avoid stereotypes and informs ways that clinicians can support parents in advocating for their children's education.
- Educators can integrate wellness skills into the school environment that inclusively support neurodiverse youth. There is evidence to support the benefits of school-based yoga programs and physical activity for neurodiverse children and adolescents. This includes improvements in self-concept, subjective well-being, executive function, academic performance, and attention.[20]

## DISCUSSION
### Mental Health Provider Well-Being

During the COVID-19, pandemic health care providers found themselves under increased demands in the work environment and their professional and personal lives, creating physical and mental health challenges. The COVID-19 pandemic has posed a great risk to the mental health of health workers. There are additional concerns for staff working with youth with intellectual disabilities. A systematic review of original research examining the mental health of health workers working with people with intellectual disabilities found that many of these workers, including nurses, physiotherapists, health care assistants, social care workers, and personal caregivers, reported they had poor mental health including stress, anxiety, and depression.[21]

Anxiety and stress have essentially become public health issues and require a system-of-care approach for recovery, treatment, and prevention. Before the pandemic there was an increased demand for mental health providers, specifically, child and adolescent psychiatrists were exiguous.[22] With even fewer clinicians available today, there has been increased attention on strategies that rely on peer[23] and community health care workers.[24] Current studies specific to the pandemic align with the results of a review of the impact of natural disasters suggesting that the youths will need positive social experiences and, in some cases, psychological interventions and treatment to restore emotional equilibrium in the months and years ahead.[25] Because of the shortage of individual providers, clinicians may need to cultivate more system- and structurally-based approaches, and community-based or partnered approaches for addressing the public health urgency of the situation. Through the pandemic, technology approaches have also helped to deliver and/or augment care.[26] Because there has been an increase in the development and availability of digital technology for mental health,[27] these digital resources and related training opportunities should be explored as additional tools for the prevention or reinforcement of clinical services.

### Schools and Primary Care

As students return to in-person learning, schools are often 'ground zero' where children are identified as needing mental health support. Because schools are uniquely positioned to provide support, they are frequently named in key federal and state policies. The American Rescue Plan Act and the Elementary and Secondary School Emergency Relief Fund, combined with other 2020 pandemic relief funds for schools, are federal responses that have been earmarked for more than $190 Billion in education and health grants available over the next 4 years, some of which can be spent on mental health.[28] The money goes to states based on their school-age population, but local school districts have decision-making authority over the lion's share of it. Ninety percent of the money allocated to states must be reallocated to school districts. Schools have wide discretion over how to spend the money if 20% or more is spent on programs to address learning loss, including summer school and after-school academic programs. Significant behavioral health resources are being provided to schools, through legislative initiatives and funding, but how to implement those effectively remains a critical concern.

Teachers have had a unique pandemic burden in managing student stress, learning new technology and COVID-19 safety protocols, and experiencing their stress, illness, and loss related to COVID-19 infection. An online survey of workers, including 135,488 teachers,[29] found that teachers reported a significantly higher prevalence of negative mental health outcomes during the COVID-19 pandemic, including anxiety and depression, when compared with health care and office workers. These additional stressors have led to job dissatisfaction and decisions to leave teaching.[30] To best support students, we need to support teachers through wellness promotion, stress management, support groups, access to behavioral health services, and other supports.

In primary care, pediatricians are tasked with assessing, triaging, and initiating treatment of common mental health concerns such as anxiety and depression.

Complicating the picture is long COVID, or long-term symptoms and consequences related to the infection after the acute stage has passed. The few studies conducted thus far provide initial evidence regarding neuropsychiatric symptoms including headaches, sleep disturbance, difficulty with concentration and memory, fatigue, and irritability,[31] With much still unknown, we anticipate a growing need for psychological support. Additionally, strategies and tools for pediatricians and their office staff to address the mental health needs of their patients can include working with schools and obtaining consultation from mental health professionals. These approaches can be framed through a tiered approach.

**Fig. 1** demonstrates a model for organizing and implementing tiered services within systems of care that integrate psychosocial and mental health treatments, promote strengthening, and enable factors across child-serving systems of care including the school setting and primary care.

### Community Networks, Support, and Healing

*Yolanda is a 17-year-old adolescent who became the primary caregiver for many of the children in her extended family. The adults in the immediate and extended family, all essential workers, contracted COVID-19 and so separated themselves from the children, while Yolanda took charge of taking care of the siblings and cousins. She helped feed them and complete their schoolwork. This was all while she struggled with her classes and schoolwork. She worried that her parents and the other adults in her life would die. She was also aware that she was important to her family, and that she had helped everyone make it through a very difficult time. During the height of the situation, the anxiety and stress were extremely distressing, but Yolanda recovered well with the support of her family and community. Community resources were critical for maintaining her well-being and contributing to her resilience despite the severity of the stress and anxiety she experienced through the pandemic. The local food hub provided food and made sure that her family had enough to eat even when her parents could not work. Her local cultural center provided traditional dancing classes and the local church offered school tutoring for her and her siblings (and the other children*

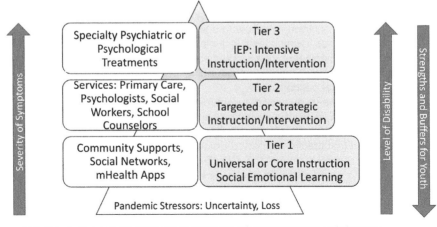

**Fig. 1.** Tiered psychological services (on *left*) and instructional supports (on *right*) for addressing youth anxiety, stress, and mental health needs in the context of pandemic stressors.

*she took care of during the height of the pandemic). They also helped Yolanda find an internship over the summer.*

Churches, synagogues, mosques, youth development organizations, cultural centers, after-school programs, and tenant and block associations are among the many community-based places and networks that can be important for supporting youths such as Yolanda and their families. These institutions and agencies are especially adept at providing social support, community building, and assistance with basic needs. A key area for mental health promotion, including addressing youth anxiety, lies in building effective community networks that bring together members of the community with the health, education, and social service professionals and organizations that serve children and families. For most communities, building effective networks means building the capacity to identify needs, assets, and potential resources. Strategies that can be particularly helpful in community settings include building capacity for mental health through partnerships across child-serving systems. In addition, offering training on mental health interventions across community networks is essential.

## SUMMARY

Social and system-based approaches are important for complementing mental health services and for addressing escalating anxiety and other mental health needs. We also need creative solutions for supporting the increased mental health services demands exacerbated during the pandemic. Although community-level interventions to combat structural racism and reduce population-level risk are sorely needed, many youths will also continue to require treatment services for anxiety. Schools are important centering environments for implementing tiered interventions. Nurturing responsive relationships with adult caregivers across community settings has been consistently identified for fostering resilience.[32] Teachers, parents, and community leaders must be supported to provide a multi-tiered and public health approach to care. Substantial structural, community, school, family, and individual level resources can help mitigate the long-term impact of the COVID-19 pandemic on child and adolescent mental health, and on children's psychosocial and educational outcomes.

## CLINICS CARE POINTS

---

To address the impact of the pandemic on anxiety disorders for youth, it is important to implement a tiered clinical, educational, and public health approach, including the following.

Clinical Services in Primary Care and Specialty Care
- Establishing methods of screening to identify children, youth, and families who may be experiencing anxiety, and identifying patient groups in need of services.
- Using integrated and collaborative care models in primary care that include case management, behavioral health, and psychiatry consultation as needed.
- Providing grief counseling for youth who have lost caregivers and other important adults including educators.
- Digital delivery of prevention and evidence-based treatments should be explored to help with broader reach and access to care.

School-Based Care from Clinical, Nursing, and Educational Staff
- Collaborating with school-based mental health professionals who provide direct support to students who are potentially at risk for emotional issues can help to implement screening processes in health centers and for referring students as appropriate to psychological support services and/or basic needs.

- Working with school nurses, who often encounter and identify when students are experiencing situations that are triggers for stress and anxiety.
- Supporting teachers and school staff in their experiences of anxiety and stress.
- Promoting student success by developing and implementing Section 504 plans, the health portion of Special Education IEP, and the Individualized Healthcare Plan.
- Promoting and practicing emotional regulation skills in schools—including supporting and contributing to implementing evidence-based programs and curricula in schools, which include strategies such as mindfulness, yoga, the arts, meditation, deep breathing, relaxation, and exercising for students and staff. Mindfulness and other wellness apps may be useful for older students.
- Identifying how earlier school closure might still be contributing to increased anxiety and loneliness in young people and child stress, sadness, frustration, indiscipline, and hyperactivity as they continue to adapt to the school setting.[33]
- Implementing evidence-based interventions including school-based cognitive behavioral therapy that are effective in decreasing anxiety symptoms and in sustaining improvements post treatment.

Community/Public Health Supports
- Engaging with community networks and social groups, churches, and other community resources as part of the continuum of care and for cultural responsiveness.
  ○ Promoting opportunities for positive relationships and positive environment
  ○ Helping meet families' basic needs
  ○ Fostering strong parent–child relationships
  ○ Promoting parents' and other caregivers' self-care
  ○ Tapping into cultural strengths, family experiences, and stories that promote families' well-being
- Remembering that resources that help with basic needs and address social determinants of mental health are best cultivated through community networks and work across child and family serving systems.

## DISCLOSURE

The authors have nothing to disclose.

## FUNDING

NIMH Grant U01 MH131827-01 awarded to authors Dr L.R. Fortuna and M.A. Porche.

## REFERENCES

1. Fortuna LR, Tolou-Shams M, Robles-Ramamurthy B, et al. Inequity and the disproportionate impact of COVID-19 on communities of color in the United States: the need for a trauma-informed social justice response. Psychol Trauma 2020;12(5):443–5.
2. Leeb RT, Bitsko RH, Radhakrishnan L, et al. Mental health-related emergency department visits among children aged <18 years during the COVID-19 pandemic - United States, January 1-October 17, 2020. MMWR Morb Mortal Wkly Rep 2020;69(45):1675–80.
3. Mercado MC, Holland K, Leemis RW, et al. Trends in emergency department visits for nonfatal self-inflicted injuries among youth aged 10 to 24 years in the United States, 2001-2015. JAMA 2017;318(19):1931–3.
4. Sharma M, Aggarwal S, Madaan P, et al. Impact of COVID-19 pandemic on sleep in children and adolescents: a systematic review and meta-analysis. Sleep Med 2021;84:259–67.

5. Racine N, McArthur BA, Cooke JE, et al. Global prevalence of depressive and anxiety symptoms in children and adolescents during COVID-19: a meta-analysis. JAMA Pediatr 2021;175(11):1142–50.

6. Terin H, Açıkel SB, Yılmaz MM, et al. The effects of anxiety about their parents getting COVID-19 infection on children's mental health. Eur J Pediatr 2022;1-7. https://doi.org/10.1007/s00431-022-04660-z.

7. Hagan MJ, Roubinov DR, Cordeiro A, et al. Young children's traumatic stress reactions to the COVID-19 pandemic: the long reach of mothers' adverse childhood experiences. J Affect Disord 2022;318:130–8.

8. Washburn M, Yu M, LaBrenz C, et al. The impacts of COVID-19 on LGBTQ+ foster youth alumni. Child Abuse Negl 2022;133:105866.

9. Gee GC, Morey BN, Bacong AM, et al. Considerations of racism and data equity among asian Americans, native hawaiians, and pacific islanders in the context of COVID-19. Curr Epidemiol Rep 2022;9(2):77–86.

10. Andrasik MP, Maunakea AK, Oseso L, et al. Awakening: the unveiling of historically unaddressed social inequities during the COVID-19 Pandemic in the United States. Infect Dis Clin North Am 2022;36(2):295–308.

11. Hillis SD, Unwin HJT, Chen Y, et al. Global minimum estimates of children affected by COVID-19-associated orphanhood and deaths of caregivers: a modelling study. Lancet 2021;398(10298):391–402.

12. California department of public health (2022). COVID-19 age, race and ethnicity data. Available at: https://www.cdph.ca.gov/Programs/CID/DCDC/Pages/COVID-19/Age-Race-Ethnicity.aspx.

13. Önder A, Sürer Adanır A, İşleyen Z, et al. Evaluation of long-term psychopathology and sleep quality in children and adolescents who presented to a university pandemic clinic with possible COVID-19 symptoms. Psychol Trauma 2022. https://doi.org/10.1037/tra0001387.

14. Spencer AE, Oblath R, Dayal R, et al. Changes in psychosocial functioning among urban, school-age children during the COVID-19 pandemic. Child Adolesc Psychiatry Ment Health 2021;15(1):73.

15. Englander E. Bullying, cyberbullying, anxiety, and depression in a sample of youth during the Coronavirus pandemic. Pediatr Rep 2021;13(3):546–51.

16. Gibbs KD, Jones JT, LaMark W, et al. Coping during the COVID-19 pandemic among young adults experiencing homelessness and unstable housing: a qualitative study. Public Health Nurs; 2022. https://doi.org/10.1111/phn.13136.

17. García-Lara RA, Gómez-Urquiza JL, Membrive-Jiménez MJ, et al. Anxiety, distress and stress among patients with diabetes during COVID-19 pandemic: a systematic review and meta-analysis. J Pers Med 2022;12(9). https://doi.org/10.3390/jpm12091412.

18. Delpino FM, da Silva CN, Jerônimo JS, et al. Prevalence of anxiety during the COVID-19 pandemic: a systematic review and meta-analysis of over 2 million people. J Affect Disord 2022;318:272–82.

19. Murphy A, Pinkerton LM, Bruckner E, et al. The impact of the novel Coronavirus disease 2019 on therapy service delivery for children with disabilities. J Pediatr 2021;231:168–77.e161.

20. Hart N, Fawkner S, Niven A, et al. Scoping review of yoga in schools: mental health and cognitive outcomes in both neurotypical and neurodiverse youth populations. Children 2022;9(6). https://doi.org/10.3390/children9060849.

21. Chen Y, Allen AP, Fallon M, et al. The challenges of mental health of staff working with people with intellectual disabilities during COVID-19–A systematic review.

J Intellect Disabil 2022. https://doi.org/10.1177/17446295221136231. 17446295221136231.

22. Findling RL, Stepanova E. The workforce shortage of child and adolescent psychiatrists: is it time for a different approach? J Am Acad Child Adolesc Psychiatry 2018;57(5):300–1.

23. Lee JB, DeFrank G, Gaipa J, et al. Applying a global perspective to school-based health centers in New York City. Ann Glob Health 2017;83(5–6):803–7.

24. Nelson EL, Zhang E, Punt SE, et al. Leveraging community health workers in extending pediatric telebehavioral health care in rural communities: evaluation design and methods. Fam Syst Health 2022;40(4):566–71.

25. Makwana N. Disaster and its impact on mental health: a narrative review. J Family Med Prim Care 2019;8(10):3090–5.

26. Psihogios AM, Stiles-Shields C, Neary M. The Needle in the haystack: identifying credible mobile health apps for pediatric populations during a pandemic and beyond. J Pediatr Psychol 2020;45(10):1106–13.

27. Sorkin DH, Janio EA, Eikey EV, et al. Rise in use of digital mental health tools and technologies in the United States during the COVID-19 pandemic: survey study. J Med Internet Res 2021;23(4):e26994.

28. National Conference of State Legislatures, Elementary and secondary school emergency relief fund tracker, Available at: https://www.ncsl.org/ncsl-in-dc/standing-committees/education/cares-act-elementary-and-secondary-school-emergency-relief-fund-tracker.aspx#relief-fund-table, 2022. Accessed November 19, 2022.

29. Kush JM, Badillo-Goicoechea E, Musci RJ, et al. Teacher mental health during the COVID-19 pandemic: informing policies to support teacher well-being and effective teaching practices. arXiv 2021. Available at: https://arxiv.org/pdf/2109.01547.pdf.

30. Gillani A, Dierst-Davies R, Lee S, et al. Teachers' dissatisfaction during the COVID-19 pandemic: factors contributing to a desire to leave the profession. Front Psychol 2022;13:940718.

31. Fainardi V, Meoli A, Chiopris G, et al. Long COVID in children and adolescents. Life 2022;12(2). https://doi.org/10.3390/life12020285.

32. Komro KA, Flay BR, Biglan A. Creating nurturing environments: a science-based framework for promoting child health and development within high-poverty neighborhoods. Clin Child Fam Psychol Rev 2011;14(2):111–34.

33. McMaughan DJ, Rhoads KE, Davis C, et al. COVID-19 related experiences among college students with and without disabilities: psychosocial impacts, supports, and virtual learning environments. Front Public Health 2021;9:782793.

# Cognitive Behavioral Therapy for Children and Adolescents with Anxiety Disorders

Jordan T. Stiede, MS[a],*, Erika S. Trent, MA[b],
Andres G. Viana, PhD[b], Andrew G. Guzick, PhD[a],
Eric A. Storch, PhD[a], Jonathan Hershfield, LCMFT[c]

## KEYWORDS

- Anxiety disorders • Children • Adolescents • Cognitive behavioral therapy • CBT
- Exposure • Case vignette

## KEY POINTS

- Cognitive behavioral therapy (CBT) is an empirically supported psychotherapeutic treatment of childhood anxiety disorders.
- Exposure therapy is the active component underlying the efficacy of CBT for childhood anxiety disorders.
- Clinicians using CBT for childhood anxiety disorders should incorporate a thorough assessment, case conceptualization, and treatment plan that adapts to the needs of all patients.

Anxiety disorders—such as specific phobias, generalized anxiety disorder, social phobia, and separation anxiety disorder—are the most common class of psychiatric conditions among children and adolescents, with estimated lifetime prevalence rates between 15% and 30% before adulthood.[1,2] Comorbidity among different anxiety disorders in youth is high,[3] and comorbid mood and externalizing disorders are also common.[4] Further, children and adolescents with anxiety disorders often experience significant functional impairment in educational, social, and familial domains, which lead to continued impairment in adulthood and increased economic burden.[1,5] The distress and impairment experienced by youth with anxiety disorders underscores the need for evidence-based interventions for these conditions. As reviewed below,

[a] Baylor College of Medicine, One Baylor Plaza, MS:350, Houston, TX 77030, USA; [b] University of Houston, 4849 Calhoun Road, Room 373, Houston, TX 77204, USA; [c] Sheppard Pratt, 6501 North Charles Street, Baltimore, MD 21204, USA
* Corresponding author.
*E-mail address:* jordan.stiede@bcm.edu

Child Adolesc Psychiatric Clin N Am 32 (2023) 543–558
https://doi.org/10.1016/j.chc.2022.12.001
1056-4993/23/© 2022 Elsevier Inc. All rights reserved.

cognitive behavioral therapy (CBT) has strong theoretic foundations, comprises core treatment components informed by theory and practice, and has substantial research support that highlight it as the gold standard treatment of childhood anxiety disorders.

## COGNITIVE BEHAVIORAL MODEL OF CHILDHOOD ANXIETY

The cognitive behavioral model of child anxiety describes anxiety as a tripartite construct consisting of physiologic, cognitive, and behavioral components.[6] Maladaptive cognitive patterns (eg, excessive worry, dysfunctional beliefs, obsessions) lead to the subjective experience of anxiety, which prompts maladaptive behaviors intended to reduce such anxiety (eg, avoidance, reassurance-seeking).[7] Physiologic arousal (eg, somatic symptoms) plays an important role in this process, wherein a child's physiologic arousal can trigger maladaptive thoughts that contribute to anxiety (eg, "My heart is beating fast, which means something is wrong"). Both theory and empirical evidence underscore the following cognitive and behavioral factors that precipitate and maintain child anxiety.

### Cognitive Factors

*Theories of cognitive processing* propose that cognitive biases contribute to the development and maintenance of childhood anxiety disorders.[8] First, children with anxiety disorders attend more heavily toward threatening information than neutral or positive information (ie, *attention biases*).[9] Second, children with anxiety disorders are predisposed to making negative or threatening interpretations of neutral or ambiguous stimuli (ie, *interpretation biases*). Greater levels of interpretation biases are associated with more severe anxiety symptoms,[10] especially when the content of ambiguous stimuli matches the anxiety subtype.[11] Interpretation biases are also stable over time and predict changes in anxiety.[12] Third, children with anxiety disorders are more likely to encode and recall threatening information over neutral or positive information (ie, *memory biases*).[13] These cognitive biases independently and additively contribute to anxiety problems in youth.[14]

The *expectancy model* of anxiety[15] posits that fear and avoidance are a function of one's expectations of, and sensitivity toward, a feared outcome. Anxiety sensitivity— the predisposition to interpret physical, cognitive, and social consequences of anxiety as threatening (eg, temperature changes, mind-racing, or other people noticing one's anxious responses)—is a cognitive factor that contributes to the development and maintenance of anxiety disorders in youth.[15,16] Anxiety sensitivity is associated with anxiety symptom severity in children and adolescents,[17] and youth with anxiety disorders report greater levels of anxiety sensitivity than nonanxious youth.[18] Anxiety sensitivity precedes and prospectively predicts anxiety symptoms across time,[19] further highlighting its contribution to the development of anxiety disorders.

### Behavioral Factors

Behavioral factors also play a significant role in reinforcing problematic anxiety. *Learning theory*[20] proposes that anxiety develops through several learning-related pathways, including aversive classic conditioning, observational learning or modeling, and information transmission.[21] When a neutral stimulus is paired with an aversive event, that neutral stimulus becomes capable of eliciting an anxiety response—a process known as aversive classic conditioning. For example, a child bitten by a dog may pair dogs (ie, neutral stimulus) with being bitten (ie, aversive event); as a result, the child generalizes their fear to all dogs, and thus any dog may elicit a phobic response. Children can also acquire fears vicariously through observational learning. A child who observes their parents' trepidation at approaching a new group of people may indirectly learn that such social encounters are dangerous, which can contribute to the development of social anxiety symptoms. Finally, children can acquire fears indirectly although verbal information received from others.[22]

Once fear learning has been established, avoidance behaviors maintain this learned fear. When children with anxiety disorders encounter a feared stimulus, and consequently experience anxiety, their instinctive response is to avoid this feared stimulus. Such avoidance provides temporary relief from anxiety and thus is negatively reinforced (ie, more likely to occur again). However, when children repeatedly undergo this process, they learn to think that the feared stimulus is in fact dangerous, and that they are incapable of handling the anxiety it provokes. Over time, anxious responses can become entrenched and increasingly severe.

## CORE TREATMENT ELEMENTS OF COGNITIVE BEHAVIORAL THERAPY FOR CHILDHOOD ANXIETY

Although some CBT programs for anxiety are disorder-specific (eg, Social Effectiveness Therapy for Children),[23] CBT programs have typically adopted a broad approach that targets a range of anxiety disorders (eg, Coping Cat).[24] Although detailing individual CBT programs is outside the scope of this review, an overview of the core treatment elements commonly shared across treatment programs is offered.[6,25]

### Psychoeducation

At the beginning of treatment, children and caregivers are provided psychoeducation about the nature of anxiety, anxiety disorders, the CBT model, and treatment details. An emphasis is placed on developing rapport with children and their parents in the first session because therapeutic alliance predicts positive treatment outcomes.[26] They are taught that anxiety is a normal response to perceived threats and serves an evolutionary purpose of keeping us safe. Anxiety disorders, however, are characterized by anxiety that is out of proportion to the actual situation and interferes with the child's day-to-day functioning (eg, a "faulty fire alarm").[24] Psychoeducation about anxiety disorders is shared to normalize the child's experience. An overview of the CBT model is presented, with a focus on the interactions between the child's physiologic sensations, thoughts, behaviors, and feelings. Finally, details of the treatment are outlined to set clear expectations and explain the rationale behind treatment.

### Anxiety Management Strategies

#### Emotional awareness training

The goal of emotional awareness training is for children to recognize somatic, behavioral, and cognitive cues of anxiety so that they use other anxiety management techniques more effectively. Children are taught strategies to recognize their anxiety, distinguish anxiety from other feelings, and use the Subjective Units of Distress Scale (SUDS) to rate anxiety severity, which is often rated from 0 (no anxiety) to 10 (maximum anxiety).

#### Relaxation training

Given the role of physiologic arousal in anxiety, relaxation training is commonly included in CBT programs. Diaphragmatic breathing exercises and progressive muscle relaxation may be taught to decrease physiologic arousal. However, recent research suggests that relaxation training may be a less central component of CBT for childhood anxiety disorders.[27]

### Problem-solving

Children are taught to problem-solve anxiety-provoking situations using a step-by-step process: identify the problem, generate multiple solutions, evaluate the costs and benefits of each solution, choose and implement the best solution, and assess the outcomes. Typically, solutions generated during this process include variants of avoidance behaviors or "approach behaviors" (ie, facing the feared situation). Children learn to evaluate the pros and cons of these behaviors, in favor of choosing approach behaviors.

### Cognitive restructuring

Consistent with cognitive theories of childhood anxiety disorders, children are taught to identify maladaptive cognitions that contribute to their anxiety and balance these with more adaptive thoughts. To help generate alternative thoughts, children systematically ask themselves a series of questions to assess and challenge overestimation of threat (eg, "How likely is the worst-case scenario?") and overestimation of negative consequences (eg, "How bad would it actually be?"). Children may be assigned a thought log for in-between sessions, in which they record situations that triggered anxiety, automatic negative thoughts, alternative thoughts, changes in SUDS, and their behavioral responses.

### Exposure

Exposure is the key active ingredient in CBT for childhood anxiety disorders.[28] Exposure techniques are based on extinction learning principles, or that repeated presentations of a feared stimulus without a negative outcome would result in extinction of a fear response.[27,29] Recently, the *inhibitory model of learning* has been proposed to explain the process of change during exposures. The inhibitory model of learning argues that, rather than unlearning their fear, through exposure to their feared situation across diverse contexts, children learn new information (eg, "that spider probably will not bite me, and even if it does, I will be able to handle it") that inhibits the fear (eg, "That spider is going to bite me and that would be really bad!").[30]

Children and clinicians collaboratively develop an exposure hierarchy, which lists a series of feared situations in order of the child-perceived difficulty. Exposures can be imaginal (an exposure involving the imagination, such as writing a story or drawing a picture), in vivo (an exposure done while interacting with the actual feared situation), or a combination of the 2. Although determining exposures is a collaborative process, clinicians must ensure that the child's core fear is being targeted. The first exposure chosen should be one that the therapist expects the child can reasonably handle, such that it is likely to be successful and provide the child a mastery experience. Mastery can be enhanced by practicing the same exposure several times to test whether the feared outcome occurs and by showing children that they can tolerate the distress that they previously perceived as unbearable. To facilitate engagement, clinicians can also propose exposure tasks that youth may find enjoyable, such as having children order food from their favorite restaurant if they have social anxiety.

Habituation-based exposures are typically conducted in a graduated fashion, from easier exposures to harder exposures. Although this may be more palatable for the child, it is not necessary for positive outcomes, assuming the child is willing to attempt exposures that evoke different levels of anxiety. The child and clinician may instead choose to move between easier and harder tasks or combine exposures in creative ways; this approach may improve outcomes by facilitating generalization of inhibitory learning.[31] That said, for children who are reluctant to try more difficult exposures, progressing from easier to more difficult is one strategy that may help facilitate engagement.

Clinicians monitor child-reported SUDS throughout exposures. Habituation-based models of exposure recommend a common rule-of-thumb that an exposure continues until the child reports at least a 50% reduction in SUDS from baseline, to ensure that habituation has occurred. Inhibitory learning models of exposure, however, recommend that exposures only need to continue until the child's expectation (eg, that something bad will happen) is violated and inhibitory learning occurs.[31] Regardless of the exposure duration, clinicians must ensure children are not using maladaptive coping strategies, both overt (eg, looking away from the feared stimulus) and covert (eg, mentally disengaging). To ensure children are practicing and generalizing their learning to other situations, exposure exercises are given as homework, and a reward program can be used to reinforce exposure homework completion.

### Relapse Prevention

Near the end of treatment, clinician, children, and caregivers consider how children will handle anxiety-provoking situations in the future. Termination occurs *not* when the child is able to tolerate situations facilitated by the clinician but rather when the child becomes adept at generalizing their skills to various situations independently. Following termination, "booster sessions" may also be offered at increasingly wide intervals, to ensure therapeutic gains are maintained posttreatment.

### RESEARCH SUPPORT FOR COGNITIVE BEHAVIORAL THERAPY FOR CHILDHOOD ANXIETY

CBT—exposures in particular—is the gold standard for treating anxiety disorders in children, as supported by empirical evidence.[25,32–35] Randomized controlled trials (RCTs) demonstrate its efficacy, with recovery rates posttreatment ranging between 47% and 66%[35] and response rates ranging between 57% and 60%.[36–38] CBT for childhood anxiety disorders also shows acceptability and safety, with no adverse effects and lower dropout rates than pharmacotherapy or pill placebo.[34]

### Comparisons with Waitlist Control

Meta-analyses consistently show that CBT outperforms waitlist or no treatment controls in terms of improvement in primary anxiety symptoms.[34,39] CBT is more than 4 times more likely to increase remission and treatment response than waitlist or no treatment.[34] Brief, intensive, and concentrated versions of CBT also outperform waitlist controls at posttreatment.[32]

### Comparisons with Active Treatment

Evidence of the superiority of CBT to other active treatments is promising. A meta-analysis found that CBT outperformed attention control (eg, psychoeducation for family members, relaxation, therapist support).[39] Although this meta-analysis found that CBT did not significantly differ from treatment-as-usual, there was significant heterogeneity between trials,[39] which indicates that these results should be interpreted with caution. Brief, intensive, and concentrated CBT outperform attention control (eg, education/support, nondirective therapy) at posttreatment but do not significantly differ from other active treatment conditions (eg, eye movement desensitization reprocessing therapy).[32] With regard to pharmacotherapy, CBT outperforms fluoxetine alone and sertraline alone, and the combination of CBT and sertraline outperforms either treatment alone as well as placebo.[34] Finally, a meta-analysis examining the effect CBT for childhood anxiety on secondary outcomes found that, in comparison to active control (eg, another treatment, self-monitoring, attention placebo, treatment-as-usual), CBT led to greater improvements in depressive symptoms and general functioning.[40]

### Key Ingredients

Although typical CBT protocols begin with anxiety management strategies (ie, emotion awareness, relaxation training, cognitive restructuring), recent dismantling studies suggest that *exposure* is the key ingredient contributing to positive treatment outcomes.[28,41] Anxiety management strategies alone are not associated with improvements in anxiety symptoms and may even be negatively associated with improvements in functioning.[28,41] In the seminal Child/Adolescent Anxiety Multimodal Study, the introduction of exposure and cognitive restructuring accelerated children's improvement in symptoms; in contrast, the introduction of relaxation techniques had little impact.[42] Further, more time devoted to difficult exposures (rather than easy or moderate) and increased child compliance and mastery within exposure sessions has been linked to better outcomes.[43] Relatedly, introduction of cognitive skills may *slow down* treatment progress.[44] A meta-analysis of RCTs comparing CBT conditions to no-treatment control found that more in-session exposure was associated with larger effect sizes (ie, larger difference between CBT condition and no-treatment control), and inclusion of relaxation training was associated with smaller pretreatment to posttreatment effect sizes.[27]

### Family Involvement in Treatment

Family accommodation (ie, parents modify their behavior to help children avoid/decrease distress from anxiety) has been linked to increased symptom severity, impairment, and worse treatment outcomes for childhood anxiety disorders; therefore, several CBT programs have included parents in treatment.[45,46] Past studies have shown mixed results regarding the increased efficacy of including parents in child anxiety treatment[45,47]; however, these studies may not have emphasized certain types of family involvement (eg, parental involvement focused on contingency management).[48] In contrast, when family involvement specifically targets parental accommodation, as has been the case in obsessive-compulsive disorder (OCD), it seems that including families bolsters outcomes.[49] Accordingly, stand-alone parent-based treatments aimed at decreasing family accommodation have shown noninferiority to individual child CBT among children with non-OCD anxiety disorders,[50] although comparison to family-based CBT is needed. Further, a meta-analysis that compared family CBT to child-only CBT found that parent–child interventions were most effective in treating anxiety disorders in children.[51] Parental involvement may be more important for girls, younger children of either sex, and children with anxiety comorbid with ADHD.[52,53] Overall, parental involvement is likely an important element of CBT for childhood anxiety disorders.

### Innovation in Cognitive Behavioral Therapy Delivery

Recent CBT research has examined digital mental health interventions to improve access and efficiency of treatment.[54] A meta-analysis of the effectiveness of telehealth versus face-to-face CBT interventions for anxiety disorders in youth and adults found no differences in anxiety symptom reduction, therapist-reported or client-reported working alliance, or client satisfaction between the 2 treatment-delivery modalities.[55] In the studies reviewed, participants had a primary diagnosis of OCD or generalized anxiety disorder, so future research is needed to generalize these findings to all anxiety disorders. Additionally, a meta-analysis of computer-based programs that deliver CBT for youth anxiety, such as BRAVE[56] and Woebot.[57] found that computer-based CBT yielded similar effects compared with active treatment controls (ie, face-to-face

CBT or treatment as usual). Of the 24 studies in the meta-analysis, 10 interventions were self-guided, whereas 14 were guided by a therapist or researcher, which included telephone and/or email contact with participants, chat sessions, or face-to-face guidance during module completion. Methodological limitations in this literature, such as primarily using self-report measures for outcome data and inappropriate handling of missing data, necessitate additional research.[58] Further, several studies have demonstrated improvements in anxiety symptoms after virtual reality exposure therapy (VRET).[59] Gutiérrez-Maldonado and colleagues[60] (2009) showed better treatment outcomes for children in VRET compared with wait-list control, whereas St-Jacques and colleagues[61] (2010) demonstrated similar outcomes between VRET and CBT-based in vivo exposure. However, future controlled trials with larger sample sizes are needed.[59] Finally, mobile apps are another tool that could be used as adjuncts to CBT treatment to help monitor homework compliance and guide exposure implementation. Anxiety Coach and SmartCat are 2 mobile apps that have demonstrated preliminary effectiveness as adjuncts to treatment.[62,63]

### Predictors of Treatment Outcomes

Identifying predictors of treatment outcomes inform efforts to personalize CBT for childhood anxiety disorders. Poorer treatment outcomes are predicted by greater anxiety severity at baseline, comorbid externalizing symptoms/disorders, and a primary diagnosis of social anxiety disorder.[64] Comorbid depression, parental psychopathology, and parental anxiety may also predict poor treatment outcomes but this evidence is less consistent.[64] Other predictors of poorer treatment outcomes for anxiety-disordered children undergoing CBT have included female gender[65] and higher levels of caregiver strain.[66]

### Practice Guidelines

Consistent with empirical evidence, the American Academy of Child and Adolescent Psychiatry's Clinical Practice Guidelines[33] provides a Level 1 recommendation (ie, the strongest recommendation) for CBT in treating children and adolescents with social anxiety, generalized anxiety, separation anxiety, panic disorder, and specific phobia.[33] Similarly, based on a review of 111 treatment outcome studies, the Society for Clinical Child and Adolescent Psychology's practice guidelines identify CBT as a "well-established" evidence-based treatment (ie, the strongest level of empirical support) for youth with anxiety disorders.[25]

### Limitations

Although extensive, the literature of RCTs for CBT in treating childhood anxiety disorders is limited by inconsistent or limited reporting of outcome measures, long-term effects of CBT, and clinically relevant variables (eg, demographic information).[34,35] Further, relatively few RCTs include children outside the 7 to 14-year age range, compare CBT with active treatment conditions, examine inpatient or intensive outpatient settings, assess for adverse effects, or examine adaptations of CBT (eg, technology-assisted CBT, parent-based CBT).[34,35] Finally, given that RCTs are commonly conducted in controlled settings with highly trained and closely supervised therapists, less is known about reproducibility of these outcomes in routine care.[35]

### CASE VIGNETTE

Sarah was a 13-year-old girl who presented for treatment with her mother because of worries related to completing school assignments and being late for events, and anxiety associated with eating in front of others and speaking with unfamiliar adults.[a] When completing homework, Sarah wanted her parents in the same room to respond to her reassurance-seeking questions regarding schoolwork. In addition, Sarah worried about being late to school and other activities, such as basketball practice. Further, Sarah struggled with eating in front of people because she feared judgment. Instead of eating lunch at school, she would eat small snacks throughout the day when others were not watching. Finally, she never ordered food for herself at restaurants, and at stores, she asked her mother to go to self-checkout to avoid talking with store clerks.

After a comprehensive evaluation, Sarah was diagnosed with generalized anxiety disorder and social anxiety disorder. A family-based CBT treatment plan was implemented, which included an initial assessment of symptoms, functional impairment, and family accommodation. Sarah was hesitant to speak with the therapist during the initial session, so most of the first session was focused on building rapport by playing a game and discussing her hobbies. Sarah and her mother were also provided with psychoeducation, which included an explanation of the development and maintenance of anxiety symptoms and the impacts of avoidance and reassurance seeking. Further, the therapist discussed the CBT treatment model using developmentally appropriate language. A motivational reward program was implemented, in which Sarah earned tokens for attending sessions, completing out-of-session homework, and participating in sessions.

In subsequent sessions, Sarah and her mother developed an exposure hierarchy with the therapist, which included a list of potential exposure exercises that Sarah rated on a 0 to 10 SUDS rating scale (**Table 1**). Sarah started with easier exposure exercises, with most exposures implemented in session before being completed for homework. For instance, Sarah ate in front of the therapist in session before completing her at-home exposure of eating in front of her family at dinner. The therapist also introduced a thought log (**Table 2**), in which Sarah tracked the triggers, thoughts, and behaviors associated with her anxiety symptoms. She was taught how to identify anxious thoughts and replace them with more realistic alternative thoughts.

Most of the treatment sessions involved the following format: (1) review exposure homework from the previous week, (2) discuss the thought log from the previous week (for situations in which Sarah struggled to develop more realistic counter thoughts, the therapist used collaborative questioning to help generate alternative thoughts), and (3) complete an in-session exposure exercise. During exposures, Sarah understood not to use her cognitive restructuring techniques, and the therapist reminded her to focus on the feared situation. Throughout treatment, the therapist encouraged Sarah's mother to coach Sarah during the in-session exposure exercises to help prepare them for exposure practice at home. The therapist also talked with Sarah's mother about the importance of not accommodating at home (eg, leaving for school and basketball practice early, providing Sarah with reassurance about schoolwork, ordering for her at restaurants).

However, as the exposure exercises became more challenging, Sarah's parents were hesitant to complete certain exposures, such as mom not helping Sarah with her homework and showing up to school 5 minutes late. A parent-only session was scheduled to explore how parents' anxiety may be related to hesitancy in completing the more challenging assignments. Parents reported that they felt guilty because not

---

[a] This case was based on the combination of several children with anxiety disorders that were treated in our clinical work. It was intended to show how CBT is administered in practice. The case is not based on a specific patient.

**Table 1**
**Sample hierarchy for a 13-year-old girl with generalized anxiety disorder and social anxiety disorder**

| Exposure Exercise | 0–10 Rating |
| --- | --- |
| Show up late to basketball practice | 9 |
| Eat messy food at school lunch | 9 |
| Turn in school homework assignment without every question completed | 9 |
| Eat messy food at family dinner | 7 |
| Show up late to school | 7 |
| Eat safe food at school lunch | 7 |
| Parents do not check homework assignment before turning it in | 7 |
| Complete homework/study for test alone (first for a few minutes, then gradually increase the amount of time) | 5–7 |
| Order for self at a sit-down restaurant | 6 |
| Eat messy food in front of therapist | 5 |
| Write a worry script about doing poorly on a test at school | 5 |
| Write a worry script about showing up late to school/basketball practice | 5 |
| Show up 5 min late to therapy session | 5 |
| Show up to school/basketball practice right as it starts instead of 15 min early | 5 |
| Order for self at a fast food restaurant without parent present | 5 |
| Turn in a therapy homework assignment without every question completed | 4 |
| Eat safe food at family dinner | 4 |
| Call businesses to ask them questions about their products | 4 |
| Eat safe food in front of therapist | 4 |
| Order for self at a fast food restaurant with parent present | 4 |
| Show up to therapy session right as it starts instead of 15 min early | 2 |

accommodating Sarah's requests in these situations led to distress and increased anxiety. Psychoeducation related to maintenance of anxiety symptoms was reviewed, and the therapist discussed how these accommodations can help reduce Sarah's anxiety and distress in the short term but often lead to more problems in the long term. The therapist also reviewed Sarah's progress in treatment, which was partially associated with her parents decreasing their reassurance and accommodations in different situations.

As treatment progressed, Sarah's anxiety symptoms gradually decreased, and she avoided fewer situations at school and home. This led to less functional impairment in school, social, and familial domains. At the end of treatment, Sarah was able to eat lunch with her friends, complete schoolwork independently, and communicate with adults in social settings. Sarah faced her feared situations that she had previously avoided, and she discovered that her feared outcomes did not occur during the exposure exercises. Toward the end of treatment, sessions were spaced 2 to 3 weeks apart, and relapse prevention was discussed with Sarah and her parents. The therapist reviewed the techniques Sarah learned in treatment and helped prepare her in the event future increases in anxiety symptoms occur.

## DISCUSSION

Anxiety disorders are frequently diagnosed in children and adolescents and can lead to impairment in multiple domains.[1,5] CBT is the gold standard treatment of childhood

**Table 2**
**Sample thought log for 13-year-old girl with generalized anxiety disorder and social anxiety disorder**

| Situation/Trigger | Thought | Emotion (0–10) | Behavior |
|---|---|---|---|
| Studying for my math test | I am going to fail the math test and get an F in the class | Anxious (7) | I asked my mom to help me study more for the test |
| In the car on the way to basketball practice, and we were only going to get there 5 min early | Coach is going to be upset that I am late and the whole team is going to stare at me when I walk in | Anxious (5) | I kept asking my dad to drive faster. I also asked him multiple times how many minutes until we get to practice |
| I ordered for myself at McDonalds | The McDonalds worker is going to laugh at me because I messed up the order | Anxious (4) | I did not make eye contact with the worker when I said my order |
| My friend saw me eating a granola bar in between classes | My friend is going to make fun of me | Anxious (7) | I stopped eating the granola bar |

anxiety disorders, with support from empirical evidence and practice guidelines.[25,33,35] Further, dismantling studies have shown that exposures are a core component of CBT for childhood anxiety disorders as anxiety management strategies alone are not associated with improvements in anxiety symptoms.[28,41] The section below reviews several important components regarding delivery of CBT for childhood anxiety disorders and discusses ways to overcome challenges associated with treatment.

### Importance of Exposures

As detailed above, exposures is a key ingredient for positive treatment outcomes in CBT for childhood anxiety disorders.[28,41,44] However, it has been found that therapists who treat children with anxiety disorders rarely used exposures because of unsubstantiated negative beliefs related to the safety, tolerability, and ethicality of exposures.[67,68] Other techniques, such as thought stopping and replacing negative thoughts with positive distraction, were used more often. This is unfortunate because such strategies may lead to avoidance of anxiety, which prolongs therapy and decreases treatment effectiveness.[69] Further, when exposures *were* delivered in treatment, they were typically patient self-directed instead of therapist-assisted, which tends to be less useful.[68] Fortunately, negative clinician beliefs related to exposures are amendable. Didactic trainings for therapists that include experiential learning and patient testimonials related to exposures have been shown to decrease these negative beliefs.[70] Dissemination of CBT treatment should continue to emphasize the rationale for and safety of exposures to clinicians.

### Addressing Clinical Complexities

Children and adolescents with anxiety disorders typically have comorbid psychiatric conditions, such as other anxiety, mood, and externalizing disorders.[3,4] These comorbidities often lead to additional complexities and challenges; therefore, thorough assessment, case conceptualization, and treatment planning are critical for best treatment outcomes. Clinicians should assess how comorbidities may affect treatment and consider whether to treat comorbidities simultaneously or sequentially to the primary anxiety disorder. Weisz and colleagues[71] (2012) indicated that incorporating free-standing modules from other evidence-based treatments for comorbid conditions may lead to enhanced outcomes. CBT for youth anxiety has also been adapted for certain conditions, such as autism spectrum disorder. Behavioral Interventions for Anxiety in Children with Autism, which includes core CBT and modules for social skills, disruptive behaviors in school, and OCD-specific behaviors, has led to moderate treatment effect sizes.[72,73]

Additionally, clinicians should adapt CBT treatment depending on the age of the child or adolescent. For instance, CBT with preadolescents should include increased parental involvement, with developmentally appropriate child psychoeducation and behavior management skills training for parents. Clinicians also must consider the unique developmental needs of adolescents and tailor treatment accordingly. Further, several programs have been developed for young children[74] and adolescents with anxiety[75] that tailor to their specific needs.

### Recommendations for Clinicians

CBT is the most well-established treatment of children and adolescents with anxiety disorders, with support from a strong literature base that demonstrates significant improvements in anxiety symptoms and impairment after treatment. Based on the literature presented above, the following recommendations regarding anxiety disorder treatment of youth are offered:

- Use a multimethod, multi-informant assessment to develop a case conceptualization and treatment plan designed to fit the needs of the diverse population of youth with anxiety disorders.
- Exposure exercises tailored to the child or adolescent's presenting concern should be a core component of treatment.
- Evaluate for possible clinical complexities and developmental needs when personalizing CBT for youth with anxiety.

### CLINICS CARE POINTS

- At the beginning of treatment, do not assume that standard CBT will be effective for each child; assess for possible clinical complexities or developmental needs that may need to be addressed in treatment.
- When completing exposures with youth, remind them to focus on the feared situation and avoid providing reassurance.
- When developing an exposure hierarchy, include feared situations with a varied degree of child-perceived difficulty and avoid only including exposures with high or low levels of difficulty.

### DISCLOSURE

Production of this article was supported by a grant from the Eunice Kennedy Shriver National Institute of Child Health & Human Development of the National Institutes of Health under Award Number P50HD103555 for use of the Clinical, United States and Translational Core facilities. The content is solely the responsibility of the authors and does not necessarily represent the official views of the National Institutes of Health, United States. J.T. Stiede and E.S. Trent have no disclosures to report. A.G.

Viana receives funding from the National Institute on Alcohol Abuse and Alcoholism, United States and honoraria from Springer and Elsevier for editorial work. A.G. Guzick receives research funding from the Ream Foundation/Misophonia Research Fund and the Texas Higher Education Coordinating Board. E.A. Storch reports receiving research funding to his institution from the Ream Foundation, International OCD Foundation, United States, and NIH, United States. He is a consultant for Brainsway and Biohaven Pharmaceuticals. He owns stock less than US$5000 in NView. He receives book royalties from Elsevier, Wiley, Oxford, American Psychological Association, Guildford, Springer, and Jessica Kingsley. J. Hershfield reports receiving book royalties from New Harbinger Publications, Inc.

## REFERENCES

1. Copeland WE, Angold A, Shanahan L, et al. Longitudinal patterns of anxiety from childhood to adulthood: the Great Smoky Mountains study. J Am Acad Child Adolesc Psychiatry 2014;53(1):21–33.
2. Kessler RC, Berglund P, Demler O, et al. Lifetime prevalence and age-of-onset distributions of DSM-IV disorders in the National Comorbidity Survey Replication. Arch Gen Psychiatry 2005;62:593–602.
3. Leyfer O, Gallo KP, Cooper-Vince C, et al. Patterns and predictors of comorbidity of DSM-IV anxiety disorders in a clinical sample of children and adolescents. J Anxiety Disord 2013;27(3):306–11.
4. Merikangas KR, Jian-ping H, Burstein M, et al. Lifetime prevalence of mental disorders in US adolescents: results from the National Comorbidity Study-Adolescent Supplement. J Am Acad Child Adolesc Psychiatry 2010;49(10): 980–9.
5. Langley AK, Bergman RL, McCracken J, et al. Impairment in childhood anxiety disorders: preliminary examination of the child anxiety impact scale–parent version. J Child Adolesc Psychopharmacol 2004;14(1):105–14.
6. Albano AM, Kendall PC. Cognitive behavioural therapy for children and adolescents with anxiety disorders: clinical research advances. Int Rev Psychiatry 2002;14(2):129–34.
7. Rapee RM, Schniering CA, Hudson JL. Anxiety disorders during childhood and adolescence: origins and treatment. Annu Rev Clin Psychol 2009;5:311–41.
8. Vasey MW, MacLeod C. Information-processing factors in childhood anxiety: a review and developmental perspective. In: Vasey MW, Dadds MR, editors. The developmental psychopathology of anxiety. London: Oxford University Press, Inc; 2001. p. 253–77.
9. Dudeney J, Sharpe L, Hunt C. Attentional bias towards threatening stimuli in children with anxiety: a meta-analysis. Clin Psychol Rev 2015;40:66–75.
10. Trent ES, Viana AG, Raines EM, et al. Interpretation biases and childhood anxiety: the moderating role of parasympathetic nervous system reactivity. J Abnorm Child Psychol 2020;48(3):419–33.
11. Stuijfzand S, Creswell C, Field AP, et al. Research review: is anxiety associated with negative interpretations of ambiguity in children and adolescents? A systematic review and meta-analysis. J Child Psychol Psychiatry 2018;59(11):1127–42.
12. Creswell C, O'Connor TG. Interpretation bias and anxiety in childhood: stability, specificity and longitudinal associations. Behav Cogn Psychother 2011;39(2): 191–204.
13. Dalgleish T, Taghavi R, Neshat-Doost H, et al. Patterns of processing bias for emotional information across clinical disorders: a comparison of attention,

memory, and prospective cognition in children and adolescents with depression, generalized anxiety, and posttraumatic stress disorder. J Clin Child Adolesc Psychol 2003;32(1):10–21.

14. Watts SE, Weems CF. Associations among selective attention, memory bias, cognitive errors and symptoms of anxiety in youth. J Abnorm Child Psychol 2006;34(6):838–49.

15. Taylor S, Koch WJ, Woody S, et al. Anxiety sensitivity and depression: how are they related? J Abnorm Psychol 1996;105(3):474–9.

16. Reiss S. Expectancy model of fear, anxiety, and panic. Clin Psychol Rev 1991; 11(2):141–53.

17. Viana AG, Trent ES, Raines EM, et al. Childhood anxiety sensitivity, fear downregulation, and anxious behaviors: vagal suppression as a moderator of risk. Emotion 2021;21(2):430–41.

18. Noël VA, Francis SE. A meta-analytic review of the role of child anxiety sensitivity in child anxiety. J Abnorm Child Psychol 2011;39(5):721–33.

19. Schmidt NB, Keough ME, Mitchell MA, et al. Anxiety sensitivity: prospective prediction of anxiety among early adolescents. J Anxiety Disord 2010;24(5):503–8.

20. Rachman S. The conditioning theory of fearacquisition: a critical examination. Behav Res Ther 1977;15(5):375–87.

21. Mineka S, Oehlberg K. The relevance of recent developments in classical conditioning to understanding the etiology and maintenance of anxiety disorders. Acta Psychol (Amst) 2008;127(3):567–80.

22. Muris P. The pathogenesis of childhood anxiety disorders: considerations from a developmental psychopathology perspective. Int J Behav Dev 2006;30(1):5–11.

23. Beidel DC, Turner SM, Morris TL. Behavioral treatment of childhood social phobia. J Consult Clin Psychol 2000;68(6):1072–80.

24. Kendall PC, Hedtke KA. Cognitive-behavioral therapy for anxious children: therapist manual. Ardmore: PA:Workbook Publishing; 2006.

25. Higa-McMillan CK, Francis SE, Rith-Najarian L, et al. Evidence base update: 50 years of research on treatment for child and adolescent anxiety. J Clin Child Adolesc Psychol 2016;45(2):91–113.

26. Liber JM, McLeod BD, Van Widenfelt BM, et al. Examining the relation between the therapeutic alliance, treatment adherence, and outcome of cognitive behavioral therapy for children with anxiety disorders. Behav Ther 2010;41(2):172–86.

27. Whiteside SP, Sim LA, Morrow AS, et al. A meta-analysis to guide the enhancement of CBT for childhood anxiety: exposure over anxiety management. Clin Child Fam Psychol Rev 2020;23(1):102–21.

28. Voort JLV, Svecova J, Jacobson AB, et al. A retrospective examination of the similarity between clinical practice and manualized treatment for childhood anxiety disorders. Cogn Behav Pract 2010;17(3):322–8.

29. Guzick AG, Schweissing E, Tendler A, et al. Do exposure therapy processes impact the efficacy of deep TMS for obsessive-compulsive disorder? J Obsessive Compuls Relat Disord 2022;35:100756.

30. Craske MG, Treanor M, Conway CC, et al. Maximizing exposure therapy: an inhibitory learning approach. Behav Res Ther 2014;58:10–23.

31. McGuire JF, Storch EA. An inhibitory learning approach to cognitive-behavioral therapy for children and adolescents. Cogn Behav Pract 2019;26(1):214–24.

32. Öst LG, Ollendick TH. Brief, intensive and concentrated cognitive behavioral treatments for anxiety disorders in children: a systematic review and meta-analysis. Behav Res Ther 2017;97:134–45.

33. Walter HJ, Bukstein OG, Abright AR, et al. Clinical practice guideline for the assessment and treatment of children and adolescents with anxiety disorders. J Am Acad Child Adolesc Psychiatry 2020;59(10):1107–24.
34. Wang Z, Whiteside SP, Sim L, et al. Comparative effectiveness and safety of cognitive behavioral therapy and pharmacotherapy for childhood anxiety disorders: a systematic review and meta-analysis. JAMA Pediatr 2017;171(11):1049–56.
35. Warwick H, Reardon T, Cooper P, et al. Complete recovery from anxiety disorders following cognitive behavior therapy in children and adolescents: a meta-analysis. Clin Psychol Rev 2017;52:77–91.
36. Bilek E, Tomlinson RC, Whiteman AS, et al. Exposure-focused CBT outperforms relaxation-based control in an RCT of treatment for child and adolescent anxiety. J Clin Child Adolesc Psychol 2022;51(4):410–8.
37. Kendall PC, Peterman JS. CBT for adolescents with anxiety: mature yet still developing. Am J Psychiatry 2015;172(6):519–30.
38. Walkup JT, Albano AM, Piacentini J, et al. Cognitive behavioral therapy, sertraline, or a combination in childhood anxiety. N Engl J Med 2008;359(26):2753–66.
39. Sigurvinsdóttir AL, Jensínudóttir KB, Baldvinsdóttir KD, et al. Effectiveness of cognitive behavioral therapy (CBT) for child and adolescent anxiety disorders across different CBT modalities and comparisons: a systematic review and meta-analysis. Nord J Psychiatry 2020;74(3):168–80.
40. Kreuze L, Pijnenborg G, de Jonge Y, et al. Cognitive-behavior therapy for children and adolescents with anxiety disorders: a meta-analysis of secondary outcomes. J Anxiety Disord 2018;60:43–57.
41. McGuire JF, Piacentini J, Lewin AB, et al. A meta-analysis of cognitive behavior therapy and medication for child obsessive-compulsive disorder: moderators of treatment efficacy, response, and remission. Depress Anxiety 2015;32(8):580–93.
42. Peris TS, Compton SN, Kendall PC, et al. Trajectories of change in youth anxiety during cognitive—behavior therapy. J Consult Clin Psychol 2015;83(2):239.
43. Peris TS, Caporino NE, O'Rourke S, et al. Therapist-reported features of exposure tasks that predict differential treatment outcomes for youth with anxiety. J Am Acad Child Adolesc Psychiatry 2017;56(12):1043–52.
44. Guzick AG, Schneider SC, Kendall PC, et al. Change during cognitive and exposure phases of cognitive–behavioral therapy for autistic youth with anxiety disorders. J Consult Clin Psychol 2022;90(9):709–14.
45. Barmish AJ, Kendall PC. Should parents be co-clients in cognitive-behavioral therapy for anxious youth? J Clin Child Adolesc Psychol 2005;34(3):569–81.
46. Lebowitz ER, Scharfstein LA, Jones J. Comparing family accommodation in pediatric obsessive-compulsive disorder, anxiety disorders, and nonanxious children. Depress Anxiety 2014;31(12):1018–25.
47. Reynolds S, Wilson C, Austin J, et al. Effects of psychotherapy for anxiety in children and adolescents: a meta-analytic review. Clin Psychol Rev 2012;32(4):251–62.
48. Manassis K, Lee TC, Bennett K, et al. Types of parental involvement in CBT with anxious youth: a preliminary meta-analysis. J Consult Clin Psychol 2014;82(6):1163–72.
49. Guzick AG, Cooke DL, Gage N, et al. CBT-plus: a meta-analysis of cognitive behavioral therapy augmentation strategies for obsessive-compulsive disorder. J Obsessive Compuls Relat Disord 2018;19:6–14.
50. Lebowitz ER, Marin C, Martino A, et al. Parent-based treatment as efficacious as cognitive-behavioral therapy for childhood anxiety: a randomized noninferiority

study of supportive parenting for anxious childhood emotions. J Am Acad Child Adolesc Psychiatry 2020;59(3):362–72.

51. Brendel KE, Maynard BR. Child–parent interventions for childhood anxiety disorders: a systematic review and meta-analysis. Res Soc Work Pract 2014;24(3): 287–95.

52. Barrett PM, Dadds MR, Rapee RM. Family treatment of childhood anxiety: a controlled trial. J Consult Clin Psychol 1996;64:333–42.

53. Maric M, van Steensel FJA, Bogels SM. Parental involvement in CBT for anxiety-disordered youth revisited: family CBT outperforms child CBT in the long term for children with comorbid ADHD symptoms. J Atten Disord 2015;22(5):506–14.

54. Khanna MS, Carper M. Digital mental health interventions for child and adolescent anxiety. Cogn Behav Pract 2022;29(1):60–8.

55. Krzyżaniak N, Greenwood H, Scott A, et al. The effectiveness of telehealth versus face to face interventions for anxiety disorders: a systematic review and meta-analysis. J Telemed Telecare 2021. https://doi.org/10.1177/1357633X211053738.

56. Waite P, Marshall T, Creswell C. A randomized controlled trial of internet-delivered cognitive behaviour therapy for adolescent anxiety disorders in a routine clinical care setting with and without parent sessions. Child Adolesc Ment Health 2019; 24(3):242–50.

57. Fitzpatrick KK, Darcy A, Vierhile M. Delivering cognitive behavior therapy to young adults with symptoms of depression and anxiety using a fully automated conversational agent (Woebot): a randomized controlled trial. JMIR Ment Health 2017;4(2):e19.

58. Christ C, Schouten MJ, Blankers M, et al. Internet and computer-based cognitive behavioral therapy for anxiety and depression in adolescents and young adults: systematic review and meta-analysis. J Med Internet Res 2020;22(9):1–20.

59. Kothgassner OD, Felnhofer A. Lack of research on efficacy of virtual reality exposure therapy (VRET) for anxiety disorders in children and adolescents. Neuropsychiatr 2021;35(2):68–75.

60. Gutiérrez-Maldonado J, Magallón-Neri E, Rus-Calafell M, et al. Virtual reality exposure therapy for school phobia. Anu Psicol 2009;40(2):223–36.

61. St-Jacques J, Bouchard S, Bélanger C. Is virtual reality effective to motivate and raise interest in phobic children toward therapy? A clinical trial study of in vivo within virtuo versus in vivo only treatment exposure. J Clin Psychiatry 2010; 71(7):924–31.

62. Silk JS, Pramana G, Sequeira SL, et al. Using a smartphone app and clinician portal to enhance brief cognitive behavioral therapy for childhood anxiety disorders. Behav Ther 2020;51(1):69–84.

63. Whiteside SP. Mobile device-based applications for childhood anxiety disorders. J Child Adolesc Psychopharmacol 2016;26(3):246–51.

64. Knight A, McLellan L, Jones M, et al. Pre-treatment predictors of outcome in childhood anxiety disorders: a systematic review. Psychopathol Rev 2014;1(1): 77–129.

65. Hudson JL, Lester KJ, Lewis CM, et al. Predicting outcomes following cognitive behaviour therapy in child anxiety disorders: the influence of genetic, demographic and clinical information. J Child Psychol Psychiatry 2013;54(10): 1086–94.

66. Compton SN, Peris TS, Almirall D, et al. Predictors and moderators of treatment response in childhood anxiety disorders: results from the CAMS trial. J Consult Clin Psychol 2014;82(2):212.

67. Schneider SC, Knott L, Cepeda SL, et al. Serious negative consequences associated with exposure and response prevention for obsessive-compulsive disorder: a survey of therapist attitudes and experiences. Depress Anxiety 2020; 37(5):418–28.

68. Whiteside SP, Deacon BJ, Benito K, et al. Factors associated with practitioners' use of exposure therapy for childhood anxiety disorders. J Anxiety Disord 2016;40:29–36.

69. Whiteside SP, Ale CM, Young B, et al. The feasibility of improving CBT for childhood anxiety disorders through a dismantling study. Behav Res Ther 2015; 73:83–9.

70. Farrell NR, Kemp JJ, Blakey SM, et al. Targeting clinician concerns about exposure therapy: a pilot study comparing standard vs. enhanced training. Behav Res Ther 2016;85:53–9.

71. Weisz JR, Chorpita BF, Palinkas LA, et al. Testing standard and modular designs for psychotherapy treating depression, anxiety, and conduct problems in youth: a randomized effectiveness trial. Arch Gen Psychiatry 2012;69(3):274–82.

72. Ung D, Selles R, Small BJ, et al. A systematic review and meta-analysis of cognitive-behavioral therapy for anxiety in youth with high-functioning autism spectrum disorders. Child Psychiatry Hum Dev 2015;46(4):533–47.

73. Wood JJ, Ehrenreich-May J, Alessandri M, et al. Cognitive behavioral therapy for early adolescents with autism spectrum disorders and clinical anxiety: a randomized, controlled trial. Behav Ther 2015;46(1):7–19.

74. Hirshfeld-Becker DR, Masek B, Henin A, et al. Cognitive behavioral therapy for 4- to 7-year-old children with anxiety disorders: a randomized clinical trial. J Consult Clin Psychol 2010;78:498.

75. Zakarin EB, Albano AM. The Launching Early Adults Program: overview of the cognitive behavioral and developmental launching emerging adults program model and implementation in a faculty practice. J Am Acad Child Adolesc Psychiatry 2016;55:72.

# Psychodynamic Formulation and Psychodynamic Psychotherapy for Pediatric Anxiety Disorders

Michael Shapiro, MD

## KEYWORDS

• Psychodynamic • Formulation • Treatment • Anxiety • Pediatric

## KEY POINTS

- Psychodynamic formulation of pediatric anxiety can help clinicians view symptoms in a biopsychosocial context influenced by development.
- The psychodynamic formulation can help the clinician select the most appropriate treatment for the patient and family.
- Psychodynamic psychotherapy is an evidence-based treatment of pediatric anxiety disorders.
- Psychodynamic therapy can be manualized and used as a short- or long-term treatment.

## INTRODUCTION

Anxiety disorders are the most common psychiatric conditions that occur across the lifespan.[1,2] Untreated anxiety disorders in childhood or adolescence place young people at risk of developing comorbid mood disorders, substance use, academic/vocational underachievement, and suicidal thoughts and attempts.[1] The assessment of childhood anxiety should involve determining whether the anxiety is expected and proportionate in the associated context or developmental challenge. Children develop typical fears and worries that are appropriate on a developmental level, such as stranger anxiety in infants and toddlers, fears of monsters around bedtime in preschool years, and worries about social status and performance in adolescence.[1] A disorder would be marked by severity that greatly impairs day-to-day functioning or is out of proportion to the child's developmental level. A psychodynamic or psychoanalytic viewpoint would help frame the anxiety symptoms in an appropriate developmental context, which is imperative in working with young people, and a rationale for

Department of Psychiatry, University of Florida, 1149 Newell Drive, Suite L4-100, Gainesville, FL 32610, USA
E-mail address: mshapiro@ufl.edu

Child Adolesc Psychiatric Clin N Am 32 (2023) 559–572
https://doi.org/10.1016/j.chc.2022.11.001
1056-4993/23/© 2022 Elsevier Inc. All rights reserved.

**childpsych.theclinics.com**

maintaining psychodynamic concepts as an integral part of child psychiatry.[3] Given the prevalence of impairment associated with pediatric anxiety disorders, advancing multiple evidence-based treatments for anxiety provides more options for patients, families, and clinicians through which to achieve improvement; psychodynamic psychotherapy is one of these options.

## HISTORY OF PSYCHODYNAMIC APPROACHES TO UNDERSTANDING PEDIATRIC ANXIETY

Before selective serotonin reuptake inhibitors (SSRIs) and cognitive-behavioral therapy (CBT), psychodynamic or psychoanalytic psychotherapy was the mainstay of treatment of childhood anxiety disorders.[4] Dating back to Sigmund Freud's publication in 1909 of 5-year-old "Little Hans" and his phobia of horses,[5] psychodynamic psychotherapy for childhood anxiety is long in the way of tradition but initially came up short regarding scientifically sound evidence. The emphasis on evidence-based medicine beginning in the 1990s led to the development of manualized treatments and a surge in randomized controlled psychotherapy trials. These trials primarily focused on CBT, which was easier to operationalize and dismantle into components than psychodynamic psychotherapy.[6] Methodological issues also plagued the perception of evidence for different psychotherapy modalities. For example, in one study comparing CBT to psychodynamic psychotherapy in the treatment of adolescents with posttraumatic stress disorder (PTSD), psychodynamic therapists were forbidden from discussing the trauma,[7] which conflicts with the standard practice of all trauma-based psychotherapies in youth. Other methodological issues that have complicated psychotherapy trials in youth include the lack of a placebo in control conditions of several studies, as "treatment-as-usual" is still treatment, and the design of short-term trials might obscure the ability to see long-term treatment gains achieved through psychodynamic psychotherapy,[8] all symptoms of a broader problem on defining what evidence-based psychotherapy really means.[9]

The focus on evidence-based medicine ultimately improved clinical trials in the early 21st century, and as a result, there is sufficient evidence showing the efficacy of psychodynamic psychotherapy,[10] including in children and adolescents. This has paved the way for several manualized, time-limited psychodynamic psychotherapies that have established efficacy for several disorders in children and adolescents, including anxiety disorders.[4,6,11–14] This evidence for psychodynamic psychotherapy in children and adolescents is buttressed by meta-analyses,[15] and systematic reviews.[16]

## DEFINITIONS

The diagnostic and statistical manual of mental disorders, fifth edition, text revision (*DSM-5-TR*) defines anxiety and fear differently although acknowledges there is overlap.[17] Anxiety is defined as the anticipation of a future threat, compared with fear, defined as an emotional response to a real or perceived imminent threat.[17] The term "fear" is warranted when it is the general consensus of objective observers that the individual's response is justified by real danger.[11] Fear responses are more often associated with surges in autonomic arousal and typically associated with fight, flight, or freeze behaviors due to an immediate danger.[17] In contrast, anxiety is generally marked more by muscle tension, vigilance, and avoidance,[17,18] in preparation for a future danger.[17] Phobias refer to fear responses to a known object and are characterized by awareness of the phobic stimuli; the response is excessive, exaggerated, or inappropriate to an objective observer and phobias are generally characterized by avoidance.[11] However, these delineations are artificial, and the terms are sometimes used interchangeably. An example of overlap would be panic attacks, which symptomatically mimic a fear response,[18] yet are classified as symptoms of anxiety disorders[17] and are also seen in non-anxiety disorders as well.[17] PTSD is marked by symptoms of vigilance and avoidance, which the DSM-5 marks as symptoms of anxiety,[17] but PTSD is not classified in the *DSM-5-TR* as an anxiety disorder[17]; phobic disorders and anxiety disorders are not separated from each other via diagnostic categories. Therefore, it may be helpful to understand all experiences along an "anxiety spectrum" related to development, evolution, psychophysiology, and psychodynamics. This article focuses on generalized anxiety disorder (GAD), separation anxiety disorder (SAD), social phobia (SP), and panic disorder (PD).

## Psychoanalytic Views

Psychoanalytic and psychodynamic theory has historically interpreted anxiety as the result of repression of some other affect or as a signal responding to threats associated with impulses of the id.[19] A traditional psychoanalytic position is that anxiety results from "threatened eruption into conscious awareness of unconscious thoughts and feelings" about which the individual feels they must avoid due to guilt, shame, or another intolerable emotional experience.[11] A contemporary psychodynamic interpretation would view anxiety as a defense mechanism that guards against and expresses a conflict between unacceptable or ambivalent intrapsychic forces.[4]

## Developmental/Evolutionary Views

From a developmental and evolutionary perspective, anxiety is adaptive and serves as an alarm system, alerting the individual to a perceived threat of danger.[4] What constitutes "danger" may be subjective and needs to be evaluated within a developmental context, such as attachment ruptures in a young child. Thus, anxiety is an innate, unconscious experience with "inborn responses" such as fight or flight,[4] driving the individual to act. Evidence suggests a "progression" from separation anxiety in young children to specific phobias or generalized anxiety in school-age children, followed by social anxiety in adolescence.[4] Neuroimaging research has pointed to a trend that in typical development, functional connectivity between brain regions such as the amygdala and medial pre-frontal cortex starts more positively in childhood, then shifts negatively during adolescence in response to fearful stimuli.[20] Other studies have corroborated such findings, particularly in cases of childhood abuse, where amygdala response to perceived threats was hyporeactive in younger children and hyperactive in adolescents.[21] It is theorized that young children must remain strongly attached to threatening caregivers to satisfy basic and attachment needs, with survival depending on the ability to reduce their responses to threats; adolescents, on the contrary, may be better able to provide for themselves and may have a more practical fight-or-flight opportunity to escape threatening situations.[21]

## Biological Views

The inhibited temperament of young children, which has been consistently associated with future risk of developing anxiety disorders, implies a biologic or genetic component contributing to a lower threshold for anxiety in response to environmental stressors.[4] Similarly, some individuals who are more prone or sensitive to a fear response; this lower threshold may predispose them to have fear mechanisms triggered by objectively minimal or innocuous stimuli.[11] Thus, in some patients, biochemical and neurophysiological mechanisms are operative, leading to some anxiety disorders being viewed as "biological" rather than psychoanalytic.[11]

### Social Learning Views

Anxiety can also be a consequence of social learning.[22] Studies have shown that observing a parent/caregiver interact in a non-anxious way with a potential threat can buffer against anxious responses in future encounters[22]; similarly, studies have shown that adults with social anxiety disorder reported more observances of their parents/caregivers to be avoidant in social situations; findings which were corroborated from the parents themselves.[22] Other avenues of social reinforcement of anxiety include direct social reinforcement, verbal instruction, and culturally transmitted rules and norms.[22]

### EVALUATION OF ANXIETY IN YOUTH: A PSYCHODYNAMIC PERSPECTIVE

Combining the theories mentioned above leads to an understanding that anxiety at its core is evolutionarily adaptive and protective, with the experience and expression of anxiety informed by genetic predispositions, temperament, biologically-based sensitivities and thresholds, learned or modeled responses based on early childhood experiences, and a tension that arises from conflicts between all of these internal forces, which may oppose each other. The Affect Phobia model is a short-term psychodynamic treatment based on Malan's Triangles of Conflict[23–25] (**Fig. 1**A), which succinctly and coherently blends this bio-psycho-social view of anxiety through the psychodynamic lens while appreciating biological and social contributions.[23]

In the affect phobia model, an "affect" is a biologically endowed set of physiologic, physical, and psychological responses that motivate people to act. The affect of fear—including the spectrum of alarm, and fright—leads to an activation of fear responses, such as running away or being hypervigilant, including fight or flight responses.[23] This view most corresponds to biological correlates of anxiety, including the propensity for oversensitivity to fear responses; from a psychodynamic viewpoint, this is most similar to the "feeling pole" of the affect phobia model, which symbolizes innate drives or feelings (id for Freudians, neurophysiology for biological psychiatrists). Inhibitory affects result in ceasing, withdrawing, or preventing action. Inhibitory affects, which include guilt and shame, function to restrict or hold back action-oriented innate feelings. Inhibitory affects are useful to moderate the response to an initial impulse so the impulse is expressed in a healthy, controlled way or are not expressed if the impulsive action would be socially prohibited. "Anxiety," which includes panic, fear paralysis, and apprehension, would inhibit behavior, thus giving the inhibitory affects its other name as the "anxiety pole."

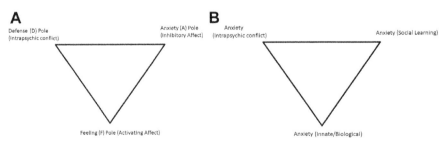

**Fig. 1.** (*A*) Malan's Triangle of Conflict (1979) adapted from Lindqvist et al (2020). (*B*) Triangle of Conflict with Anxiety serving as unconscious feeling/impulse, inhibitory anxiety, or defense mechanism.

Maladaptive patterns of affect expression develop when children are taught that there is something wrong with their inner emotional responses; this could also be that their emotional reaction is frightening to others and, therefore themselves. Importantly, many inhibitory affects are learned through early childhood experiences with parents/caregivers. Such adults use inhibitory affects such as fear, guilt, or shame to shape their children's behavior; when excessive inhibition is placed on a child's adaptive activating affects, this can lead to a phobic avoidance of that affect and that only certain expressions are allowable. The socially learned component of anxiety best correlates with what is known as the "Anxiety Pole" of affect phobia theory ("superego" for Freudians, cognitive distortions for behaviorists). We therefore can have a situation where adaptive anxiety, interpreted as the need to protect oneself and others, can be neutralized or opposed by maladaptive anxiety, including traumatic anxiety and panic. Defense mechanisms arise to manage such conflicts. As any feeling can function as a defense, it is important to recognize that anxiety can also present as a defensive affect. According to McCullough, affects that are likely to be defensive present as atypical or inappropriate for the context. Although they may be maladaptive, they can also be seen as functioning to meet the patient's needs in some way.[23] A list of "defensive behaviors" contains many examples of what may be attributed to anxiety: passivity, withdrawing, not speaking up, and avoiding eye contact (**Box 1**).[23]

Anxiety as a symptom can therefore represent any of the three poles of Malan's triangle: innate excessive biological response (Feeling), learned reaction in response to early childhood experiences (Anxiety), or a defensive affect responding to internal conflicts (Defense; **Fig 1**B). The first task of the psychodynamic formulation of anxiety is to determine whether anxiety is being experienced as a defense mechanism, as an innate but excessive/exaggerated biological process, or as something learned from early experiences that are blocking the experience of naturally occurring affect phenomenon. A psychodynamic perspective is important as the answer to this question has implications regarding treatment planning (**Fig. 2**).

---

**Box 1**
**Example of defensive anxiety**

- An adolescent had recently gone to a public event with their family, hoping to spend quality time together. Once at the event, the family split off in different directions, leaving the adolescent alone.

- The adolescent identified feeling angry at being deserted and wanted to ask their family to come back, but felt guilty about being "selfish" by exerting control over the family.

- The adolescent felt anxious and developed a panic attack, marked by shortness of breath, tachycardia, and a sensation of choking. Owing to the choking, the patient texted the rest of the family that they were having a panic attack as they were unable to vocally call to them. The family received the text messages and returned to comfort the adolescent.

- The defensive nature of the panic attack can be identified by:
  o Being inappropriate to context, where anger or disappointment would have been expected
  o Preventing the adolescent's conscious awareness/expression of the unacceptable affect– anger
  o Functioning to express the conflict by meeting the patient's need for closeness while avoiding feelings of anger and guilt

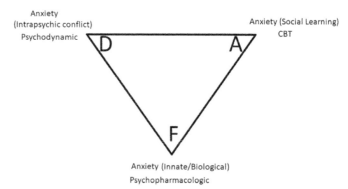

**Fig. 2.** Interpretation of Malan's Tringle of Conflict with targeted treatment interventions based on whether anxiety as a treatment focus is experienced: psychodynamic therapy when anxiety is a defense mechanism (*D*), CBT when anxiety is a learned inhibitory response (*A*), and psychopharmacology when anxiety is due to excessive innate physiologic response (*F*).

## CLINICS CARE POINTS

- A psychodynamic formulation of anxiety examines whether anxiety is experienced as:
  - an innate/excessive biological process, and may respond to medications
  - learned through early social experiences, and may respond to CBT
  - a defensive affect responding to internal conflicts and may respond to psychodynamic psychotherapy

## GUIDELINES

The American Academy of Child & Adolescent Psychiatry (AACAP) Clinical Practice Guideline for the treatment of pediatric anxiety disorders[2] includes only two treatments purported to have sufficient evidence meriting recommendation: CBT and SSRIs. In this analysis, CBT is defined as interventions that target three primary dimensions of anxiety: cognitive distortions, behavioral avoidance, and physiologic/autonomic arousal. CBT involves changing maladaptive beliefs and attitudes while using graduated exposure, processes which are learned in a social context. Medications, including SSRIs, target the biologic/physiologic "innate feeling" pole. Although the validity of the serotonin hypothesis for depression has been questioned recently,[26] serotonin may modulate of fear, worry, and stress and the associated neurocircuitry in pediatric anxiety disorders.[2,27] Despite the guideline advocating that the evaluation of anxiety leads to the development of a clinical formulation that includes "hypothesized psychological vulnerabilities," including those derived from psychodynamic theory, such as unconscious conflicts, and that treatment planning is derived from the clinical formulation, the guideline suggested insufficient information to conclude non-CBT psychotherapies that contrast with a surfeit of evidence for other psychotherapeutic interventions—including psychodynamic psychotherapy—in pediatric anxiety disorders.

## PSYCHODYNAMIC APPROACH

Psychodynamic psychotherapy has traditionally not been tailored to single diagnoses or specific symptoms[19]; instead, it focuses on core underlying processes common to various disorders, including unresolved conflicts, affect regulation, internalizing object relations, and insecure attachment.[19] This may limit the perception of its efficacy in randomized trials compared with CBT, as in such studies, CBT tends to be specifically tailored to treat anxiety, setting up unfair comparisons.[7,9,19] However, as previously discussed, anxiety may have clear psychodynamic origins in some situations, including those in which it is rooted in unconscious conflicts, and systematic study of alternatives to CBT may identify which type of intervention works best for whom.[6] Another important difference between psychodynamic psychotherapy and CBT is the delayed treatment effects that may be seen in psychodynamic psychotherapy compared with CBT. Several studies suggest that psychodynamic psychotherapy has a "sleeper effect," such that significant improvement is seen most clearly after the end of the active treatment.[8] This has important ramifications not only for patient/family treatment preference but also in evaluating the evidence of short-term trials, which may favor behavioral treatments like CBT or other symptom-focused therapies. It is theorized that psychodynamic psychotherapy, by working on internal object representations, reflective functioning, and insight and self-awareness, produces a delayed treatment response as these changes precede behavioral changes; treatments that directly modifying behavior may produce earlier improvement, especially when using behavior-specific outcomes that are common in anxiety inventories used as outcomes in most pediatric anxiety studies,[28,29] but such changes may not be as long-lasting.[8] In addition, it is possible that without addressing the core conflicts, the resolution of some symptoms may lead to the emergence of new symptoms or defense mechanisms that merely take their place.

Psychodynamic psychotherapy is distinguishable from CBT in that it focuses on understanding the unconscious meaning of anxiety symptoms.[4,6] Practically speaking, CBT addresses cognitive distortions, automatic thoughts and avoidance that produce anxiety, but psychodynamic psychotherapy examines the context and unconscious processes that originally fuel the cognitive distortions. Manualized psychodynamic therapies for anxiety have several common core principles. In addition to elements common to almost all psychotherapies—such as psychoeducation, setting treatment goals, and establishing a therapeutic alliance—psychodynamic psychotherapy for anxiety involves identifying core conflicts, focusing on warded-off affects, modifying internalized object relations, and changing defenses and avoidance.[19] The process of understanding the meaning of the symptoms verbally or acting out/in-play with younger children, reworks memories and unconscious associations to improve dysregulated attachment and promote normal reflective functioning. In psychodynamic psychotherapy with children, anxiety is viewed as being related to underlying emotional meanings of conflicts operating outside of children's awareness; when young people are able to access and better define their emotional understanding, this promotes a sense of safety and allows them to act autonomously and to be less avoidant. Psychodynamic psychotherapy is also distinguishable from CBT in that while presenting anxiety symptoms remain in therapist's focus, there is more attention paid to what is absent (the warded off against affects), who is not mentioned (past conflicts), contextual elements pointing to where vigilance and soft spots occur, and dominant themes that connect the symptoms together.

## APPLICATION

In general, the typical dynamic of pediatric anxiety involves parents who attempt to protect their child from what they perceive as frightening and overwhelming experiences and situations, leading to a situation where the child forms a symbiotic relationship with the parent by identifying with the anxiety, while also desiring and yet being fearful of separation/individuation needs that may be viewed by the parent as rejecting or dangerous.[14] In other words, the anxiety symptoms result from the need to compromise wishes for separation/individuation against the perception those wishes are unacceptable due to guilt or fear of harm befalling the child or the parent by attempting to make efforts toward separation/individuation.[4] The task of the therapist is to encourage separation and individuation and allow the child to experience aggressive and individuating behaviors and see that they do not damage the self or the other.[14] Common psychodynamic themes that underly pediatric anxiety include fear of separation/autonomy from attachment figures, difficulty experiencing/acknowledging anger, sexual or identity conflicts, and conflicted guilt and/or anger expressed as self-punishment.[4]

Child and Adolescent Anxiety Psychodynamic Psychotherapy (CAPP) is a short-term, manualized psychotherapy adapted from Panic-Focused Psychodynamic Psychotherapy (PFPP), another manualized psychodynamic psychotherapy with evidence in adults with PD.[4,6] CAPP is a transdiagnostic approach intended for children 8 to 16 years of age as a twice-weekly intervention, composed of 20 to 24 sessions divided into opening, middle, and termination phases marked by specific tasks[4–6]:

1. Opening Phase—Obtaining history, developing an alliance, theorizing tentative formulations, psychoeducation on emphasis on anxiety symptoms, and uncovering the meaning behind the symptoms
2. Middle Phase—Applies psychodynamic focus to patterns revealed through the history, provide interpretations on these patterns and possible hidden meanings, normalizing age-appropriate wishes/fantasies, encouraging self-reflection, reducing the rigidity of defensive behaviors
3. Closing Phase—Reinforce self-reflection and new flexibility, anticipate anxiety rearousal, interpret the transference, revisit with family, demonstration of new behavior patterns

CAPP also suggests common themes and conflicts prevalent among the various disorders. These will be briefly summarized.

### Generalized Anxiety Disorder

A common theme found in children and teens with GAD is the fear of losing control, and that the loss of control will lead to catastrophe and the resultant guilt and shame. The persistent anxiety can result from the emergence of unacceptable feelings or wishes that threaten maintaining control or perfectionism, and these upsetting feelings are experienced as frightening, dangerous, or disruptive. Somatization may also appear as a defense. The worry itself may function as almost a magical thinking belief that enough worrying will prevent catastrophe or bad outcomes, thus the prospect of worrying less may paradoxically be accompanied by more fear of loss of control.

### Social Anxiety Disorder

Patients with social anxiety symptoms frequently have conflicted emotional responses to attachment figures, including fear of separation and tolerating their own angry feelings. There may be a predominance of conflicted views of assertiveness and fantasies of grandiosity and exhibitionism. Symptoms, risk factors, and central dynamics may mimic those of PD and have been associated with behavioral inhibition and inhibited temperament in early childhood and in family members. Individuals with social anxiety may have a core sense of inadequacy at acting autonomously, including a sense that they may betray others, including their family, by increasing their social network, and fear that doing so will threaten existing attachment relationships. Patients then project intense anger onto others whom they perceive as rejecting.

### Separation Anxiety Disorder

Core underlying fears of abandonment of either themselves or parents speaks to ambivalence or discomfort with the level of durability in their current attachment, and inability to tolerate ambivalent feelings in relationships. Precipitants may be real or imagined threats of abandonment, including projected fears of a parent, or past traumas that threatened the attachment of either the child or the parent to the other. Therapeutic techniques will need to incorporate the inevitable threat of separation with the therapist at termination.

### Panic Disorder

Conflicted fantasies and worries about separation and autonomy are often at the core of PD. Precipitants can also be real or fantasized loss of separation, including fear of separation due to conflict anger, need for autonomy, and sexual feelings/identity.

## CURRENT EVIDENCE

Muratori and colleagues[13,16] performed a preliminary study of 14 children with SAD assigned to psychodynamic psychotherapy (ten children were assigned to treatment-as-usual) comprising 11 sessions: five with the child alone, five parent-child join sessions, and a final joint termination session. The Child Behavior Checklist (CBCL) and the Children's Global Assessment Scale (C-GAS) were assessed at baseline, at the end of active treatment at 6 months, and at 2-year follow-up. The group treated with psychodynamic psychotherapy had fewer problems and better functioning at 6 months and this superiority was still observable at 2-year follow-up. Although both groups improved during the 6-month active treatment phase,[13,16] only the psychodynamic treatment group had significant improvement at the 2-year follow-up.[8] These results support previous evidence that psychodynamic psychotherapy with young people produces a "sleeper effect" leading to continued improvement even after the end of the study period.[8]

Göttken and colleagues[12,16] evaluated manualized, short-term psychoanalytic child therapy (PaCT) in children aged 4 to 10 years with anxiety disorders. A younger age group was selected due to the perceived limitation of CBT in children who have not attained concrete operations and CBT studies yielded improvement but less remissions than expected. The treatment consisted of approximately 20 to 25 weekly psychotherapy sessions for 18 families, including parent-child, child-alone, and parent-alone appointments; 12 families served as waitlist controls before themselves receiving the intervention. Sessions focused on identifying and modifying core conflicts underlying the symptoms and family dynamics using play therapy with the children, and parent sessions every fourth session, with the therapist addressing possible unconscious meanings of the child's symptoms, aiming to uncover and work through relational themes underlying anxiety symptoms. The most common diagnoses were GAD, social anxiety and specific phobias and the study included children with comorbid depression and externalizing behaviors. Parents completed (CBCL) weekly and two-thirds of youth who completed therapy achieved remission. Impressively, remission was maintained at a 6-month follow-up visit.

Weitkamp and colleagues[14,16] compared both short-term (≤24 sessions) and long-term (≥25 sessions) psychoanalytic psychotherapy ($n = 86$) compared with minimally supportive control ($n = 35$) for children and adolescents with severe anxiety disorders. The final length of treatment was determined by clinical need, with this flexibility included due to a previous study of 25 sessions, which, although showed clinically significant and reliable improvement compared with the wait list (62% vs 8%), observed some youth appeared to have more severe symptoms and require more intense treatment.[30] Patients received twice-weekly individual therapy sessions mixed with parent sessions at a ratio of 4:1 over 3 months. Anxiety was assessed using the Screen for Child Anxiety-Related Emotional Disorders (SCARED)[31] and Quality of Life (QoL) was also assessed. In this flexible-dose model, 87% of patients completed long-term therapy (>25 sessions); the average duration of treatment was 90 sessions over 2 years. Over the initial 25 sessions, comprising the first treatment period, there were no statistically significant differences in improvement between the intervention group and the control group, as both led to significant decreases in symptoms. There was significant improvement at the end of the therapy period, gains that remained at 6-month and 12-month follow-up after therapy ended. By both patient and parent evaluation, symptoms and functioning at 6 months after treatment termination were better than at the end of treatment although patients reported greater improvement than did their parents and half of the sample met criteria for recovery/remission.

Salzer and colleagues[16,32] performed a multicenter randomized controlled trial comparing CBT and psychodynamic psychotherapy for adolescents with social anxiety disorder. Patients aged 14 to 20 years were randomized to 25 sessions of CBT ($n = 34$), psychodynamic psychotherapy ($n = 34$), or a waitlist ($n = 39$). In both CBT and psychodynamic psychotherapy arms, the 25 sessions were scheduled weekly, with some twice-weekly at the start of treatment. The Liebowitz Social Anxiety Scale for Children and Adolescents and the Social Phobia Anxiety Inventory were administered as baseline and follow-up assessments at the end of treatment, and 6- and 12-month post-treatment. Both CBT and psychodynamic psychotherapy were superior to the control condition and efficacious in reducing social anxiety symptoms, with medium-to-large effects for CBT and medium effects for psychodynamic psychotherapy; effects were stable at 12-month follow-up for both treatments.[16,32]

## SUMMARY, AND FUTURE DIRECTIONS

Psychodynamic psychotherapy is an effective treatment of pediatric anxiety disorders that can be implemented in time-limited and manualized formats and produces positive outcomes that appear to be maintained. When considering treatment of children and adolescent anxiety disorders, patient and family preference should be considered with regard to other evidence-based treatment approaches (eg, CBT, SSRIs).

There are limitations. As not all patients benefit from CBT or SSRIs,[29] not all patients will improve with psychodynamic psychotherapy.[16] Psychodynamic psychotherapy may be considered a first-choice approach for patients with at least average cognitive capacity and cognitive flexibility and both secure and insecure working models of attachment.[33] Future research should consider providing guidance on which patients or families benefit most from psychodynamic treatments compared with other treatment modalities, how to more easily and quickly detect such patients and families, and how to conceptualize the cost-benefit ratio of short-term compared with long-term psychodynamic psychotherapy for pediatric anxiety disorders. In addition to length of treatment, dose of treatment should be further studied, as previous studies of psychoanalytic psychotherapy for a variety of diagnoses and disorders suggested that younger children benefit from more intense treatment frequency compared with adolescents.[34]

This is an exciting time for psychodynamic psychotherapy. The quantity and quality of research supporting the effectiveness of psychodynamic psychotherapy has grown exponentially in the last decade,[10] and specifically the evidence for use in children and adolescents has dramatically increased.[16]

Novel delivery methods have also been studied and are proving effective, especially Internet-based psychodynamic psychotherapy.[25,35–40] Several trials have already been completed for Internet-based psychodynamic psychotherapy for adults with anxiety disorders[35–37] and for adolescents with depression.[25,38,39] These studies have suggested Internet-delivered psychodynamic psychotherapy is acceptable to patients,[37,38] and one study of 36 adults with social anxiety showed that Internet-based psychodynamic psychotherapy was preferred more often than ICBT (63.9% vs 36.1%), although without reaching statistical significance.[37] In addition to being acceptable and even preferable, Internet-based psychodynamic psychotherapy appears effective[25,35,36,38,39] and comparable in effectiveness to Internet-based CBT (ICBT) for depression and anxiety disorders.[35,37,39] One study of Internet-based group psychodynamic psychotherapy for adults showed effectiveness of anxiety and somatic disorders, particularly for social anxiety.[40] More studies for Internet-based psychodynamic psychotherapy for child and adolescent anxiety disorders is warranted.

The ability to provide high-quality care via Internet-based delivery methods was an important development In light of the paradigm shift to telemedicine during the COVID-19 pandemic.[38,40,41]

One albeit small study found that children and adolescents with anxiety disorders were particularly well-suited for video-mediated psychotherapy during the pandemic.[41] In addition, the rapid proliferation of tele-mental health may be a venue in which high-quality psychodynamic and psychoanalytic psychotherapies can be delivered to traditionally underserved populations, including racial/ethnic minorities, and those without insurance coverage or in lower socioeconomic strata.[42] We join previous calls to improve efforts at making psychodynamic and psychoanalytic psychotherapy training and delivery more inclusive, accessible, and affordable.[42–44]

## DISCLOSURE

The author has no commercial or financial conflicts of interest.

## REFERENCES

1. Strawn JR, Peris TS, Walkup JT. Anxiety disorders. In: Dulcan MK, editor. Dulcan's textbook of child and adolescent psychiatry. 3rd edition. Washington, DC: American Psychiatric Association Publishing; 2022.
2. Walter HJ, Bukstein OG, Abright AR, et al. Clinical practice guideline for the assessment and treatment of children and adolescents with anxiety disorders. J Am Acad Child Adolesc Psychiatry 2020;59(10):1107–24.
3. American Academy of Child and Adolescent Psychiatry. Policy statement: psychotherapy as a core competence of child and adolescent psychiatrist. Approved by Council January; 2014. https://www.aacap.org/aacap/Policy_Statements/2014/Psychotherapy_as_a_Core_Competence_of_Child_and_Adolescent_Psychiatrist.aspx.
4. Silver G, Shapiro T, Milrod B. Treatment of anxiety in children and adolescents: using child and adolescent anxiety psychodynamic psychotherapy. Child Adolesc Psychiatr Clin N Am 2013;22(1):83–96.
5. Ritvo RZ, Shapiro M. Chapter 6.2.5: Psychodynamic principles in practice. In: Martin B, Shapiro MA, editors. *Lewis's child and adolescent psychiatry: a*

*comprehensive textbook*. 5th edition. Philadelphia, PA: Wolters Kluwer; 2017. p. 807.

6. Preter SE, Shapiro T, Milrod B. Child and adolescent anxiety psychodynamic psychotherapy: a treatment manual. New York, NY: Oxford University Press; 2018.

7. Abbass A, Luyten P, Steinert C, et al. Bias toward psychodynamic therapy: framing the problem and working toward a solution. J Psychiatr Pract 2017; 23(5):361–5.

8. Muratori F, Picchi L, Bruni G, et al. A two-year follow-up of psychodynamic psychotherapy for internalizing disorders in children. J Am Acad Child Adolesc Psychiatry 2003;42(3):331–9.

9. Shedler J. Where is the evidence for "evidence-based" therapy? Psychiatr Clin North Am 2018;41(2):319–29.

10. Shedler J. The efficacy of psychodynamic psychotherapy. Am Psychol 2010; 65(2):98–109.

11. Gardner RA. Children with separation anxiety disorder. In: O'Brien Pilowsky, Lewis, editors. Psychotherapies with children and adolescents: adapting the psychodynamic process. Washington, DC: American Psychiatric Press, Inc; 1992. p. 3–23.

12. Göttken T, White LO, Klein AM, et al. Short-term psychoanalytic child therapy for anxious children: a pilot study. Psychotherapy (Chic) 2014;51(1):148–58.

13. Muratori F, Picchi L, Apicella F, et al. Psychodynamic psychotherapy for separation anxiety disorders in children. Depress Anxiety 2005;21(1):45–6.

14. Weitkamp K, Daniels JK, Baumeister-Duru A, et al. Wirksamkeit analytischer Psychotherapie bei Kindern und Jugendlichen mit klinischen Angstsyndromen im naturalistischen Behandlungssetting [Effectiveness of Psychoanalytic Psychotherapy for Children and Adolescents with Severe Anxiety Psychopathology in a Naturalistic Treatment Setting]. Prax Kinderpsychol Kinderpsychiatr 2019; 68(3):209–18.

15. Abbass AA, Rabung S, Leichsenring F, et al. Psychodynamic psychotherapy for children and adolescents: a meta-analysis of short-term psychodynamic models. J Am Acad Child Adolesc Psychiatry 2013;52(8):863–75 [published correction appears in J Am Acad Child Adolesc Psychiatry. 2013;52(11):1241].

16. Midgley N, Mortimer R, Cirasola A, et al. The evidence-base for psychodynamic psychotherapy with children and adolescents: a narrative synthesis. Front Psychol 2021;12:662671.

17. American Psychiatric Association. Diagnostic and statistical manual of mental disorders. 5th edition. Washington, DC: Text Revision (TR); 2022.

18. Hamm AO. Fear, anxiety, and their disorders from the perspective of psychophysiology. Psychophysiology 2020;57(2):e13474.

19. Leichsenring F, Salzer S. A unified protocol for the transdiagnostic psychodynamic treatment of anxiety disorders: an evidence-based approach. Psychotherapy (Chic) 2014;51(2):224–45.

20. Treanor M, Rosenberg BM, Craske MG. Pavlovian learning processes in pediatric anxiety disorders: a critical review. Biol Psychiatry 2021;89(7):690–6.

21. Zhu J, Lowen SB, Anderson CM, et al. Association of prepubertal and postpubertal exposure to childhood maltreatment with adult amygdala function. JAMA Psychiatry 2019;76(8):843–53.

22. Mineka S, Zinbarg R. A contemporary learning theory perspective on the etiology of anxiety disorders: it's not what you thought it was. Am Psychol 2006;61(1): 10–26.

23. McCullough L, Kuhn N, Andrews S, et al. Treating affect phobia: a manual for short-term dynamic psychotherapy. New York: The Guildford Press; 2003.

24. Malan DH. Individual psychotherapy and the science of psychodynamics. London, UK: Butterworths; 1979.

25. Lindqvist K, Mechler J, Carlbring P, et al. Affect-focused psychodynamic internet-based therapy for adolescent depression: randomized controlled trial. J Med Internet Res 2020;22(3):e18047.

26. Moncrieff J, Cooper RE, Stockmann T, et al. The serotonin theory of depression: a systematic umbrella review of the evidence. Mol Psychiatry 2022. https://doi.org/10.1038/s41380-022-01661-0 [published online ahead of print, 2022 Jul 20].

27. Lu L, Mills JA, Li H, et al. Acute neurofunctional effects of escitalopram in pediatric anxiety: a double-blind, placebo-controlled trial. J Am Acad Child Adolesc Psychiatry 2021;60(10):1309–18.

28. Piacentini J, Bennett S, Compton SN, et al. 24- and 36-week outcomes for the child/adolescent anxiety multimodal study (CAMS). J Am Acad Child Adolesc Psychiatry 2014;53(3):297–310.

29. Swan AJ, Kendall PC, Olino T, et al. Results from the child/adolescent anxiety multimodal longitudinal study (CAMELS): functional outcomes. J Consult Clin Psychol 2018;86(9):738–50.

30. Kronmüller KT, Postelnicu I, Hartmann M, et al. Zur Wirksamkeit psychodynamischer Kurzzeit- psychotherapie bei Kindern und Jugendlichen mit Angststörungen [Efficacy of psychodynamic short-term psychotherapy for children and adolescents with anxiety disorders]. Prax Kinderpsychol Kinderpsychiatr 2005;54(7):559–77.

31. Birmaher B, Khetarpal S, Brent D, et al. The screen for child anxiety related emotional disorders (SCARED): scale construction and psychometric characteristics. J Am Acad Child Adolesc Psychiatry 1997;36(4):545–53.

32. Salzer S, Stefini A, Kronmüller KT, et al. Cognitive-behavioral and psychodynamic therapy in adolescents with social anxiety disorder: a multicenter randomized controlled trial. Psychother Psychosom 2018;87(4):223–33.

33. Delgado SV, Strawn JR, Pedapati EV. Contemporary psychodynamic psychotherapy for children and adolescents: integrating intersubjectivity and neuroscience. New York: Springer; 2015.

34. Target M, Fonagy P. The efficacy of psychoanalysis for children: prediction of outcome in a developmental context. J Am Acad Child Adolesc Psychiatry 1994;33(8):1134–44.

35. Andersson G, Paxling B, Roch-Norlund P, et al. Internet-based psychodynamic versus cognitive behavioral guided self-help for generalized anxiety disorder: a randomized controlled trial. Psychother Psychosom 2012;81(6):344–55.

36. Johansson R, Hesslow T, Ljótsson B, et al. Internet-based affect-focused psychodynamic therapy for social anxiety disorder: a randomized controlled trial with 2-year follow-up. Psychotherapy (Chic) 2017;54(4):351–60.

37. Lindegaard T, Hesslow T, Nilsson M, et al. Internet-based psychodynamic therapy vs cognitive behavioural therapy for social anxiety disorder: a preference study. Internet Interv 2020;20:100316.

38. Midgley N, Guerrero-Tates B, Mortimer R, et al. The depression: online therapy study (D:OTS)-A pilot study of an internet-based psychodynamic treatment for adolescents with low mood in the UK, in the context of the COVID-19 pandemic. Int J Environ Res Public Health 2021;18(24):12993. Published 2021 Dec 9.

39. Mechler J, Lindqvist K, Carlbring P, et al. Therapist-guided internet-based psychodynamic therapy versus cognitive behavioural therapy for adolescent

depression in Sweden: a randomised, clinical, non-inferiority trial. Lancet Digit Health 2022;4(8):e594–603.

40. Wajda Z, Kapinos-Gorczyca A, Lizińczyk S, et al. Online group psychodynamic psychotherapy-The effectiveness and role of attachment-The results of a short study. Front Psychiatry 2022;13:798991.

41. Erlandsson Anette, Forsström David, Alexander Rozental, et al. Accessibility at what price? therapists' experiences of remote psychotherapy with children and adolescents during the COVID-19 pandemic. J Infant, Child, Adolesc Psychotherapy 2022. https://doi.org/10.1080/15289168.2022.2135935.

42. Mongelli F, Georgakopoulos P, Pato MT. Challenges and opportunities to meet the mental health needs of underserved and disenfranchised populations in the United States. Focus (Am Psychiatr Publ) 2020;18(1):16–24.

43. Rosenberg JM. A call for inclusiveness in the psychoanalytic community. Psychoanal Rev 2022;109(1):35–8.

44. Pacheco NE. Examining racism in psychoanalytic training: perspectives from a psychiatry resident. Psychodyn Psychiatry 2021;49(4):481–6.

# Advances in Pharmacotherapy for Pediatric Anxiety Disorders

Cassandra M. Nicotra, DO[a], Jeffrey R. Strawn, MD[a,b],*

## KEYWORDS

- Selective serotonin reuptake inhibitor (SSRI)
- Serotonin and norepinephrine reuptake inhibitor (SNRI)  • Benzodiazepine
- Buspirone  • Guanfacine  • Tricyclic antidepressant (TCA)  • Anxiety disorders
- Generalized anxiety disorder (GAD)

## KEY POINTS

- Selective serotonin reuptake inhibitors (SSRIs) are the first-line psychopharmacologic treatment for pediatric anxiety disorders.
- SSRIs and serotonin and norepinephrine reuptake inhibitors (SNRIs) differ in their tolerability.
- The risk of treatment-emergent suicidality does not differ between SSRIs, SNRIs, and placebo in pediatric patients with anxiety disorders.

| Abbreviations | |
| --- | --- |
| GAD | Generalized anxiety disorder |
| SNRI | Serotonin and norepinephrine reuptake inhibitor |
| SSRI | Selective serotonin reuptake inhibitor |
| TCA | Tricyclic antidepressant |

## INTRODUCTION

More than a dozen prospective randomized trials suggest that multiple medication classes are effective for youth with anxiety disorders. These trials focus on generalized anxiety disorder (GAD), social anxiety disorder, and separation anxiety disorder,

[a] Department of Pediatrics, Division of Child & Adolescent Psychiatry, Cincinnati Children's Hospital Medical Center, Cincinnati, OH 45267, USA; [b] Department of Psychiatry and Behavioral Neuroscience, University of Cincinnati, College of Medicine, Cincinnati, OH 45219, USA
* Corresponding author. Department of Psychiatry and Behavioral Neuroscience, University of Cincinnati, College of Medicine, Cincinnati, OH 45219.
*E-mail address:* strawnjr@uc.edu

Child Adolesc Psychiatric Clin N Am 32 (2023) 573–587
https://doi.org/10.1016/j.chc.2023.02.006
1056-4993/23/© 2023 Elsevier Inc. All rights reserved.

childpsych.theclinics.com

referred to as the "pediatric anxiety triad." These disorders are highly comorbid and have a similar response to pharmacotherapy.[1–3] This review summarizes randomized controlled trials of SSRIs, SNRIs, benzodiazepines, and other agents (**Table 1**) and reviews their tolerability, the trajectory of response, and the role of pharmacotherapy in combination with psychotherapy for treating youth with anxiety disorders.

## SELECTIVE SEROTONIN REUPTAKE INHIBITORS

Selective serotonin reuptake inhibitors (SSRIs) are the most commonly used medications for pediatric anxiety disorders.[4] As a class, SSRIs, relative to serotonin norepinephrine reuptake inhibitors (SNRIs), produce improvement early (by 2 weeks) (**Fig. 1**), and nearly half of the improvement seen by 12 weeks is evident by 4 weeks. Additionally, earlier improvement may occur in patients treated with higher SSRI doses.[5] A network meta-analysis of 22 randomized controlled trials of SSRIs and SNRIs along with tricyclic antidepressants (TCAs), benzodiazepines, 5-HT$_{1A}$ agonist (buspirone), and $\alpha_2$ agonist (guanfacine) in youth with anxiety disorders found that SSRIs were the most effective class of medications.[6]

### Escitalopram

Escitalopram, the s-enantiomer of citalopram, is a highly serotonergically-specific SSRI[7,8] and has been evaluated in two prospective double-blind, placebo-controlled trials of youth with GAD. First, forced flexible titration of escitalopram to 15 to 20 mg in adolescents with GAD (n = 26) for 8 weeks was superior to placebo (n = 25). In this study, greater improvement was seen in slower CYP2C19 metabolizers. The discontinuation rate was similar for escitalopram and placebo, and bruising was the only adverse event more common in patients receiving escitalopram versus those receiving placebo. Activation (impulsivity, irritability, restlessness, insomnia, and so forth) was associated with higher plasma escitalopram concentrations but not the absolute dose.[9] In the second study of escitalopram, children and adolescents (age 7–17 years) with GAD were treated with flexibly dosed escitalopram (n = 138; 10–20 mg/d) or placebo (n = 137) for 8 weeks. The mean change from baseline to week eight on the Pediatric Anxiety Rating Scale (PARS) of severity for GAD score was significantly greater for escitalopram than for placebo. Escitalopram was relatively well tolerated, with treatment-emergent adverse events occurring in approximately 55% of patients receiving escitalopram and 40% of those receiving placebo. No evidence of QTc prolongation was observed in either study.[10]

Finally, 1 small open-label study of flexibly-dosed citalopram (10–40 mg/d, mean dose 35 ± 7 mg/d, n = 12) in children and adolescents aged 8 to 17 years (mean age 13.4 ± 3 years) with social anxiety disorder found that 83% of youth responded based on Clinical Global Impression Improvement (CGI-I) scale. Patients and parents also reported improved social anxiety symptoms, and citalopram was well tolerated.[10]

### Fluoxetine

Birmaher and colleagues (2003) evaluated the efficacy and tolerability of fluoxetine in a fixed-dose, randomized, placebo-controlled trial of youth (age 7–17 years, N = 37) with GAD, separation anxiety disorder, and social anxiety disorder.[11] In this 12-week trial, fluoxetine was initiated at 10 mg and titrated to 20 mg daily at the end of the first week. Fluoxetine-treated patients had greater improvements on dimensional and global measures of anxiety and functioning than placebo, which was statistically significant by week nine. Fluoxetine was well tolerated[11] and a follow-up study

**Table 1**
Selected randomized controlled trials of pharmacologic interventions in pediatric anxiety disorders

| Reference | Diagnoses | Age (y) | Duration (wk) | Treatment Modalities | N | Dose Range (mg/d) | Average Dose |
|---|---|---|---|---|---|---|---|
| Strawn et al,[10] 2023 | GAD | 7-17 | 8 | Escitalopram<br>Placebo | 138<br>137 | 10-20 | Flexibly dosed |
| Strawn et al,[9] 2020 | GAD | 12-17 | 8 | Escitalopram<br>Placebo | 26<br>25 | 15-20 | Fixed dose |
| Beidel et al,[13] 2007 | SocAD | 7-17 | 12 | Fluoxetine<br>Placebo<br>SET-C | 33<br>57<br>32 | 10-40 | Fixed dose |
| Birmaher et al,[11] 2003 | GAD<br>SocAD<br>SepAD | 7-17 | 12 | Fluoxetine<br>Placebo | 37<br>37 | 20 | Fixed dose |
| Walkup et al,[1] 2008 | GAD<br>SocAD<br>SepAD | 7-17 | 12 | Sertraline<br>CBT<br>Combination<br>Placebo | 133<br>139<br>140<br>76 | 25-200<br>25-200 | 146.0 ± 60.8 mg<br>133.7 ± 59.8 mg |
| Rynn et al,[16] 2001 | GAD | 5-17 | 9 | Sertraline<br>Placebo | 11<br>11 | 50 | Fixed dose |
| Walkup et al,[22] 2001 (RUPP) | GAD<br>SocAD<br>SepAD | 6-17 | 8 | Fluvoxamine<br>Placebo | 61<br>63 | 50-300<br>Max 250 in <12 yo<br>Max 300 in adolescents | 2.9 ± 1.3 mg/kg |
| Wagner et al,[24] 2004 | SocAD | 8-17 | 16 | Paroxetine<br>Placebo | 163<br>156 | 10-50 | 24.8 mg for all patients, 21.7 mg for children, and 26.1 mg for adolescents |
| March et al,[26] 2007 | SocAD | 8-17 | 16 | Venlafaxine ER<br>Placebo | 137<br>148 | 37.5-225 | 2.6-3 mg/kg |

(continued on next page)

**Table 1
(continued)**

| Reference | Diagnoses | Age (y) | Duration (wk) | Treatment Modalities | N | Dose Range (mg/d) | Average Dose |
|---|---|---|---|---|---|---|---|
| Rynn et al,[25] 2007 | GAD | 6-17 | 8 | Study 1: Venlafaxine ER | 76 | 37.5-225 | Flexibly dosed based on weight |
| | | | | Placebo | 77 | | |
| | | | | Study 2: Venlafaxine ER | 78 | 37.5-225 | Flexibly dosed based on weight |
| | | | | Placebo | 82 | | |
| Strawn et al.,[27] 2015 | GAD SocAD SepAD | 7-17 | 10 | Duloxetine | 135 | 30-120 | Flexibly dosed |
| | | | | Placebo | 137 | | |
| Strawn et al,[37] 2017 | GAD SocAD SepAD | 6-17 | 12 | Guanfacine | 62 | 1-6 | 0.06-0.12 mg/kg for 50 kg, 3-6 mg for >50 kg |
| | | | | Placebo | 21 | | |
| Strawn et al,[34] 2018 | GAD | 6-17 | 6 | Study 1: Buspirone | 111 | 15-60 | Flexibly dosed |
| | | | | Placebo | 111 | | |
| | | | | Study 2: Buspirone | 221 | 15-60 | Fixed dose |
| | | | | Placebo | 112 | | |

*Abbreviations:* GAD, generalized anxiety disorder; SepAD, separation anxiety disorder; SET-C, Social Effectiveness Therapy for Children; SocAD, social anxiety disorder; ER, extended-release venlafaxine.

*Adapted from* Strawn, et al. Psychopharmacologic Treatments of Children and Adolescents with Anxiety Disorders. Child and Adolescent Psychiatric Clinics of North America. 2012;21(3):527-539.

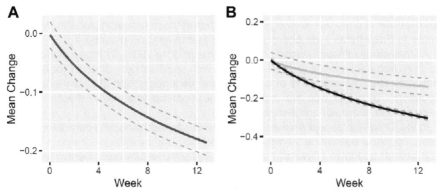

**Fig. 1.** Response trajectory in antidepressant-treated children and adolescents with DSM-5 anxiety disorders. Dotted *grey* lines represent the 95% credible interval. (*A*) Red line represents the overall standardized medication (SSRI and SNRI)-placebo mean difference over time with the best-fit model (logarithmic). (*B*) The blue line represents SSRI-placebo difference. Green line represents SNRI-placebo difference. (*Reproduced from* Strawn, et al. The impact of antidepressant dose class on treatment response in pediatric anxiety disorders: A meta-analysis. Journal of the American Academy of Child and Adolescent Psychiatry. 2018;57;4;235-244.)

suggested that fluoxetine may be effective as a maintenance treatment in children and adolescents with anxiety disorders.[12]

A double-blind, randomized trial compared Social Effectiveness Therapy for Children (SET-C), fluoxetine (forced titration 10–40 mg/d), and placebo in children and adolescents (age 7–17 years) with social anxiety disorder (Diagnostic and Statistical Manual of Mental Disorders, Fourth Edition, DSM-IV criteria). Fifty-three percent of the SET-C group no longer met diagnostic criteria (compared to 21.2% of patients treated with fluoxetine and 3.1% of those treated with placebo) after 8 weeks of treatment. SET-C and fluoxetine were superior to placebo in all outcome measures and overall functioning.[13]

Two open-label studies have evaluated fluoxetine in youth with anxiety disorders. In the first study, youth with mixed anxiety disorders (overanxious disorder/GAD, or separation anxiety disorders) who failed to respond to psychotherapy were treated with flexibly-dosed fluoxetine for up to 10 months. Birmaher and colleagues (1994) observed moderate to marked improvements in 81% of patients, and fluoxetine was well tolerated.[14] Later, Fairbanks and colleagues (1997) evaluated 16 outpatients (age 9–18 years) who failed to respond to psychotherapy and were treated with flexibly-dosed fluoxetine (5 mg daily, titrated to a maximum of 40 mg in children and 80 mg daily in adolescents).[15] Clinical improvement occurred in all patients with separation anxiety disorder (n = 10), 8 of 10 with social anxiety disorder, 3 of 5 with panic disorder, and 1 of 7 with GAD, with a mean time to improvement of 5 weeks. Fluoxetine was well tolerated, with the most frequent side effects being drowsiness, sleep problems, anorexia, nausea, and abdominal pain. In this study, patients with only 1 anxiety disorder responded to lower doses of fluoxetine than those with multiple anxiety disorders (0.49 ± 0.14 mg/kg vs 0.80 ± 0.28 mg/kg).[15]

### *Sertraline*

In a placebo-controlled trial of fixed-dose sertraline (50 mg/d), youth aged 5 to 17 years with GAD (n = 22) were treated for 9 weeks. Compared with placebo-treated youth,

Hamilton Anxiety Rating Scale (HAM-A) scores and global measures of improvement were greater in patients receiving sertraline than in those receiving placebo. No differences in side effects were observed between sertraline and placebo.[16]

A small study of flexibly-dosed sertraline (mean dose 123 ± 37 mg/d) evaluated 14 children and adolescents (age 10–17 years) with social anxiety disorder for 8 weeks. Based on CGI-I scores, 36% of patients were responders, and 29% were partial responders. Sertraline was well tolerated; the most common side effects reported were nausea, diarrhea, and headaches.[17]

In the Child/Adolescent Anxiety Multimodal Study, sertraline was compared to placebo, cognitive behavioral therapy (CBT), and their combination (sertraline + CBT) in 488 patients aged 7 to 17 years (mean age 11.8 years) over 12 weeks. Sertraline was superior to placebo, and the combination of sertraline + CBT was superior to both monotherapy and placebo. Specifically, improvement (CGI-I) scores for sertraline + CBT were greater (80.7%) than those for CBT (59.7%) or sertraline alone (54.9%). Rates of adverse events with sertraline were similar to those with placebo. However, those children who received CBT were less likely to report insomnia, fatigue, sedation, restlessness, or fidgeting than those who received sertraline.[1] Predictors of remission included younger age, nonminority status, lower baseline anxiety severity, absence of other internalizing disorders (eg, anxiety, depression), and absence of social phobia.[18] Additionally, in this study, response emerged relatively early,[19] sertraline was well tolerated,[20] and response was maintained for many youth over a 6-month follow-up period.[21]

### Fluvoxamine

Fluvoxamine was evaluated in a double-blind, placebo-controlled trial in youth with anxiety disorders (N = 128). In this study, children were treated with fluvoxamine titrated to 300 mg daily (mean dose 2.9 ± 1.3 mg/kg). Global improvement and dimensional measures of anxiety were significantly better in patients receiving fluvoxamine than in those receiving placebo. In addition, fluvoxamine was well tolerated, with only abdominal discomfort and increased motor activity occurring more frequently than it does in those who received placebo.[22] In a 6-month, open-label extension study, 94% of fluvoxamine responders maintained response, and 71% of the fluvoxamine-treated patients who had not initially responded to fluvoxamine subsequently improved.[23]

### Paroxetine

While paroxetine has been less frequently used, as it is associated with greater treatment emergent suicidality,[6] 1 large study evaluated its efficacy in pediatric anxiety disorders. In this multicenter, double-blind, placebo-controlled trial of paroxetine, Wagner and colleagues (2004) randomized 322 youth (aged 8–17 years) with social anxiety disorder.[24] They observed greater responses (by CGI-I score) in paroxetine-treated youth (n = 161) than in those receiving placebo (n = 156); response rates were 78% and 38.3%, respectively. Insomnia, decreased appetite, and vomiting were among the most common side effects, and four paroxetine-treated patients reported suicidal ideation compared to zero patients in the placebo group. Upon discontinuation, SSRI withdrawal symptoms, including nausea, dizziness, and vomiting, were experienced twice as frequently by patients treated with paroxetine compared to those who received placebo.[24]

## SELECTIVE SEROTONIN AND NOREPINEPHRINE REUPTAKE INHIBITORS

In a meta-analysis of 22 randomized controlled trials of SNRIs and SSRIs, TCAs, benzodiazepines, 5-HT$_{1A}$ agonist (buspirone), and $\alpha_2$ agonist (guanfacine) found SNRIs as a class to have a more frequent treatment response versus placebo but less so than SSRIs. Additionally, in this meta-analysis, SNRIs were the most tolerable class with statistically significantly less discontinuation due to adverse effects than other treatments.[6]

### Venlafaxine

Extended-release venlafaxine (venlafaxine ER) has been evaluated in two 8-week, randomized placebo-controlled trials involving youth with GAD aged 6 to 17 years (N = 323). Venlafaxine ER was initiated at 37.5 mg daily and was titrated based on weight. In the pooled analysis, venlafaxine ER was superior to placebo in improving scores derived from the GAD section of the Columbia Kiddie Schedule for Affective Disorders and Schizophrenia (K-SADS). Improvements on the PARS, HAM-A, and Screen for Child Anxiety Related Disorders (SCARED) parent and child scores were also statistically significant compared to placebo in 1 study but failed to reach statistical significance in the second study. Relative to other SNRIs, venlafaxine may be less tolerable; venlafaxine was also associated with more asthenia, pain, anorexia, somnolence, and weight loss than those receiving placebo.[25]

Venlafaxine ER was also evaluated in children and adolescents (age 8–17 years, n = 293) with social anxiety disorder. In this study, venlafaxine ER was initiated at 37.5 mg daily and titrated to a maximum dose based on weight over 16 weeks (dose range 112.5–225 mg). Youth receiving venlafaxine ER had a greater reduction in their symptoms than those receiving placebo (response rates 56% vs 37%, respectively). Significant weight loss was noted in several patients treated with venlafaxine ER, and three patients receiving venlafaxine ER developed suicidal ideation compared to zero patients receiving placebo.[26]

### DULOXETINE

A 10-week, randomized placebo-controlled trial of duloxetine in children and adolescents (age 7–17 years) with GAD found that duloxetine (30–120 mg daily) was superior to placebo in improving dimensional measures of anxiety (PARS severity for GAD), as well as measures of functioning, including the Children's Global Assessment Scale and response/remission based on Clinical Global Impression Severity scale score. Duloxetine was associated with weight loss and increased heart rate, and there were no differences in discontinuation rate or suicidality emergence between duloxetine and placebo.[27]

### Atomoxetine

Atomoxetine was evaluated in a placebo-controlled trial of children and adolescents (age 8–17 years) with attention-deficit/hyperactivity disorder (ADHD) and comorbid anxiety (GAD, separation anxiety disorder, and/or social anxiety disorder). Atomoxetine was initiated at 0.8 mg/kg/d for 3 days and increased to the target dose of 1.2 mg/kg/d, with a maximum dose of 1.8 mg/kg/d; treatment was continued for 12 weeks. A last observation carried forward analysis of PARS scores revealed improvement with atomoxetine versus placebo (effect size = 0.5) along with significant improvements in ADHD symptoms. Atomoxetine was generally well tolerated[28]; however, it is noteworthy that this study did not use the CYP2D6 genotype to guide dosing, which is the current recommendation.

### Benzodiazepines

Benzodiazepines, the positive allosteric modulators at gamma-aminobutyric acid-A (-GABA$_A$) receptors, vary in their affinity, time of onset, and duration of effect in adults with anxiety disorders.[29] However, despite the common use of benzodiazepines for the treatment of anxiety disorders in adults, trials of this class of medication in youth with anxiety disorders have produced mixed results. One open-label trial of 12 adolescents with overanxious disorder (the DSM-III-R forerunner of GAD) treated with alprazolam (0.5–1.5 mg/d) for 4 weeks noted significant improvements in anxiety and insomnia. Alprazolam was generally well tolerated despite some sedation, agitation, headaches, and nausea.[30] However, double-blind trials have failed to identify drug-placebo differences. A double-blind, placebo-controlled trial of alprazolam in youth aged 8 to 16 years (N = 30) with overanxious disorder found no difference between alprazolam and placebo on CGI-I; however, the study was significantly underpowered. Alprazolam was well tolerated in this study but with some reports of fatigue and dry mouth. No withdrawal symptoms were identified.[31]

One study evaluated clonazepam (up to 2 mg/d) in children (age 7–13 years) with separation anxiety disorder (n = 14) and GAD (n = 5) using a crossover design. In this study, CGI-I was observed between youth receiving clonazepam and those receiving placebo and failed to show a significant difference. Side effects were more common in those receiving clonazepam (83%) than in those receiving placebo (58%) and included drowsiness, irritability, and oppositional behavior.[32]

In a meta-analysis of 22 randomized controlled trials that included three studies of benzodiazepines,[31–33] benzodiazepines were the least effective class, and early discontinuation was more likely, specifically with clonazepam.[6]

### Buspirone

A 2018 analysis of two randomized controlled trials of buspirone, a $5HT_{1A}$ agonist, in youth aged 6 to 17 years with GAD found no significant differences in improvement between youth receiving buspirone and those receiving placebo using K-SADS as the primary outcome. In these studies, the discontinuation rate of buspirone was similar to that of SSRIs and SNRIs. Lightheadedness was the most common adverse event, consistent with adult studies.[34]

Additionally, an open-label trial of buspirone in youth with overanxious disorder found that over 6 weeks of treatment, flexibly dosed buspirone (15–30 mg/d) was associated with improvement in anxiety.[35] Subsequently, in 13 children and 12 adolescents with anxiety, Salazar and colleagues (2001) reported improvement in anxiety over 4 weeks of treatment.[36] In both open-label studies, buspirone was generally well tolerated although some patients experienced sedation, nausea, stomachaches, and headaches.

### Guanfacine

In a pilot trial, flexibly dosed extended-release guanfacine (guanfacine ER) was compared to placebo in pediatric patients aged 6 to 17 years with GAD, separation anxiety disorder, and/or social anxiety disorder (N = 83). Guanfacine was safe and tolerable compared to placebo. Guanfacine ER did not differ from placebo in scores on the PARS although statistically significant improvements were noted on global measures of severity. The most common adverse effects reported were headache, somnolence/fatigue, abdominal pain, and dizziness, consistent with its known side effect profile from pediatric ADHD and tic disorder studies.[37] Of note, in this trial, the dosing of guanfacine was relatively low and significantly below a typical dose in youth with ADHD (ie, >0.08 mg/kg).[38]

### Tricyclic Antidepressants

In recent years, TCAs have been less commonly used secondary to their side effect profiles, yet several older studies have evaluated youth with school refusal along with comorbid separation and/or social anxiety disorders. First, 35 children (age 6–14 years) were treated with flexibly dosed imipramine (100–200 mg/d). Imipramine-treated patients improved more than those who received placebo.[39] However, subsequent trials of TCAs in youth with school refusal, overanxious disorder, and separation anxiety disorder have failed to find differences between imipramine or clomipramine and placebo.[33,40] Finally, Bernstein and colleagues (2000) compared combination treatments of imipramine + CBT to placebo + CBT in 63 adolescents (mean age: 13.9 ± 3.6 years) with major depressive disorder and an anxiety disorder.[41] In this study, school attendance and clinician-rated depression significantly improved in the patients who received imipramine + CBT compared with that in those who received placebo + CBT. However, neither clinician- nor self-report measure of anxiety significantly differed between groups.[41]

### Combination of Pharmacotherapy and Psychotherapy

Psychotherapeutic treatment of youth with anxiety disorders is becoming more widely recognized as a part of the evidence-based, comprehensive treatment plan. Of the available studies of psychotherapy, most have evaluated the efficacy of CBT,[1,19,42–45] and several alternate forms of psychotherapy that are efficacious in other types of psychopathology in youth remain understudied in those with anxiety disorders (eg, interpersonal psychotherapy for adolescents, mentalization-based therapy). In general, synergistic effects of psychotherapy and psychopharmacologic interventions have been observed,[1,19,46] and current practice guidelines from the American Academy of Child & Adolescent Psychiatry recommend a multimodal treatment approach.[47]

### Tolerability of Selective Serotonin Reuptake Inhibitors and Serotonin and Norepinephrine Reuptake Inhibitor

Two meta-analyses have examined the risks of specific adverse events in children and adolescents treated with SSRIs and SNRIs.[6,48] Strawn and colleagues' 2015 meta-analysis of SSRIs and SNRIs in youth found that discontinuation due to adverse effects was similar to relative risk estimates derived from recent network meta-analyses that focused primarily on efficacy and compared multiple medication classes (eg, SSRIs, SNRIs, TCAs, benzodiazepines, $\alpha_2$ agonists).[48]

Across disorders, SSRIs are more likely to produce activation, abdominal pain, sedation/drowsiness, and adverse-effect-related discontinuation than placebo. SSRI tolerability is similar among pediatric patients with anxiety disorders and obsessive-compulsive disorder (OCD) as well as depressive disorders.[49] The relationship between SSRI dosing and exposure has received limited attention, and there are very few data concerning the discontinuation or tapering of SSRIs in children and adolescents. Several studies suggest that some SSRIs may have more adverse effects at higher doses (or in patients with greater exposure).[35] With very few exceptions, these studies do not consider variations in pharmacodynamic genes that may differentially affect side effect expression nor differences in pharmacokinetic genes that produce variation in metabolism and, thus, differences in exposure, even when patients are treated with the same dose.

### Adverse Effects

Clinical trials of antidepressants in youth rarely examine the time course of side effects, yet clinicians know that some side effects emerge early and resolve quickly (eg, activation, gastrointestinal symptoms). In contrast, other side effects are tardive (eg, weight gain) or persistent (eg, sexual dysfunction). For acutely emerging side effects, such as gastrointestinal symptoms, dynamic physiologic relationships may mitigate these effects. For example, nausea, which emerges early, may relate to acute increases in serotonergic tone, thus increasing gastrointestinal motility. The resolution of gastrointestinal side effects may relate to the desensitization of enteric serotonergic receptors.[49] Discussing the temporal course of the side effects and distinguishing between static and dynamic side effects are critical in clinical practice. Ensuring that patients are aware not only of the potential types of side effects (**Fig. 2**) but also about the tendency of some side effects to be transient is important and should be part of discussions with patients and their families prior to the initiation of pharmacotherapy. Understanding the transient nature of many side effects may improve adherence and mitigate anxiety related to treatment with antidepressant medications.

### Pharmacogenetics

Several studies have evaluated the role of pharmacogenetics in pediatric patients with anxiety and related disorders. In general, for SSRIs metabolized by CYP2C19 (ie, sertraline and escitalopram/citalopram), slower metabolizers have greater medication exposure at a given dose than faster metabolizers,[9,50,51] and escitalopram-related adverse events are more likely in slower metabolizers.[52] However, for CYP2D6-metabolized SSRIs (ie, fluoxetine, paroxetine), the evidence is less clear. Regarding pharmacogenetic testing in child and adolescent psychiatry, we recommend considering pharmacogenetic test results for genes with high levels of evidence if they are available or testing if the clinician feels that results of evidence-based genes (eg, CYP2D6, CYP2C19, HLA-A, HLA-B) would inform medication dosing or selection. This recommendation concords with the International Society of Psychiatric Genetics, which supports CYP2C19 and CYP2D6 testing for patients having had inadequate

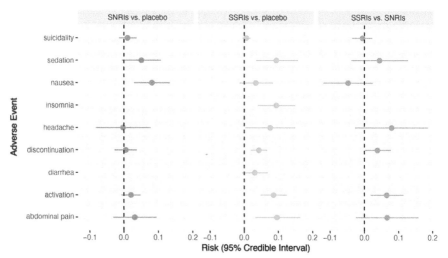

**Fig. 2.** Relative risk of antidepressant-related adverse effects (AEs), suicidality, and discontinuation secondary to adverse effects. The relative risk of each AE is shown in addition to the 95% credible interval. The large interval estimates for AE-related discontinuation and suicidality relate to the small number of occurrences relative to the number of patients leading to a skewed distribution when converting the estimated relative probabilities to the log odds scale, rather than an indication of large potential chances of those outcomes. (*Reproduced from* Mills and Strawn, Antidepressant tolerability in pediatric anxiety and obsessive compulsive disorders: A Bayesian hierarchical modeling meta-analysis. Journal of the American Academy of Child and Adolescent Psychiatry. 2020;59(11):1240-1251.)

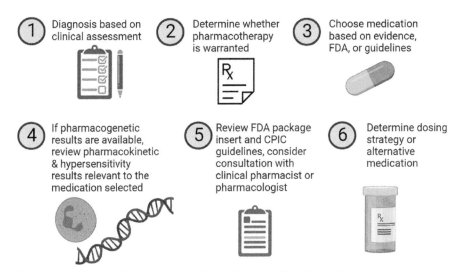

**Fig. 3.** Incorporation of pharmacogenetic testing into clinical practice. Graphic description of proposed pharmacogenetic testing approach for children and adolescents. CPIC, clinical pharmacogenetics implementation consortium. (Created with BioRender.com.)

responses to or adverse effects with antidepressants or antipsychotics.[53] Importantly, deciding whether to use a specific pharmacologic intervention should be based on thorough evaluation and available evidence from efficacy studies. Pharmacogenetic testing, when obtained, should influence dosing and alter the level of monitoring or choice of medication within the evidence-based class of medications for a given disorder (**Fig. 3**).[54,55]

## SUMMARY

In children and adolescents with anxiety disorders, double-blind, placebo-controlled trials support the efficacy of the SSRIs and SNRIs, but there are mixed results for other medication classes. SSRIs are more effective than SNRIs for anxiety symptom improvement. Additionally, SSRI + CBT produce greater benefit than SSRI monotherapy across most internalizing disorders, including anxiety disorders.[19] SSRIs and SNRIs should be initiated after a discussion with patients and families regarding the risk of potential adverse effects. Initial doses should be low and titrated slowly to minimize these effects, particularly activation syndrome. Pharmacogenetic testing can be used as a guide for dosing and monitoring strategies for selected medications.[54]

## CLINICS CARE POINTS

---

- SSRIs are the most effective pharmacotherapy for pediatric anxiety disorders and represent the first-line medication.
- In patients who have not responded to an initial SSRI, a trial of a second SSRI represents the next best step prior to a trial of an SNRI.
- Combining pharmacotherapy and psychotherapy consistently produces the best outcomes in youth with anxiety disorders.

---

## DISCLOSURE

Dr J.R. Strawn has received research support from the Yung Family Foundation, the National Institutes of Health (NIMH/NIEHS/NICHD), the National Center for Advancing Translational Sciences, the Patient Centered Outcomes Research Institute (PCORI), and Abbvie. He has received material support from Myriad Health and royalties from three texts (Springer). Dr J.R. Strawn serves as an author for *UpToDate* and an Associate Editor for *Current Psychiatry* and has provided consultation to the FDA, Cereval Therapeutics, and IntraCellular Therapies. Views expressed within this article represent those of the authors and are not intended to represent the position of NIMH, the National Institutes of Health (NIH), or the Department of Health and Human Services. Dr C.M. Nicotra has no disclosures.

## ACKNOWLEDGMENTS

This work was supported by the Yung Family Foundation, the National Institutes of Health (NICHD, R01HD098757, R01HD099775, JRS).

## REFERENCES

1. Walkup JT, Albano AM, Piacentini J, et al. Cognitive behavioral therapy, sertraline, or a combination in childhood anxiety. N Engl J Med 2008;359(26):2753–66.
2. Compton SN, Walkup JT, Albano AM, et al. Child/adolescent anxiety multimodal study (CAMS): rationale, design, and methods. Child Adolesc Psychiatry Ment Health 2010;4:1.
3. Kendall PC, Compton SN, Walkup JT, et al. Clinical characteristics of anxiety disordered youth. J Anxiety Disord 2010;24(3):360–5.
4. Bushnell GA, Compton SN, Dusetzina SB, et al. Treating pediatric anxiety: initial use of SSRIs and other antianxiety prescription medications. J Clin Psychiatry 2018;79(1).
5. Strawn JR, Mills JA, Sauley BA, et al. The impact of antidepressant dose and class on treatment response in pediatric anxiety disorders: a meta-analysis. J Am Acad Child Adolesc Psychiatry 2018;57(4):235–44.e232.
6. Dobson ET, Bloch MH, Strawn JR. Efficacy and tolerability of pharmacotherapy for pediatric anxiety disorders: a network meta-analysis. The Journal of clinical psychiatry 2019;80(1):14375.
7. Sánchez C, Bergqvist PB, Brennum LT, et al. Escitalopram, the S-(+)-enantiomer of citalopram, is a selective serotonin reuptake inhibitor with potent effects in animal models predictive of antidepressant and anxiolytic activities. Psychopharmacology (Berl) 2003;167(4):353–62.
8. Culpepper L. Escitalopram: a new SSRI for the treatment of depression in primary care. Prim Care Companion J Clin Psychiatry 2002;4(6):209–14.
9. Strawn JR, Mills JA, Schroeder H, et al. Escitalopram in adolescents with generalized anxiety disorder: a double-blind, randomized, placebo-controlled study. J Clin Psychiatry Aug 25 2020;81(5).
10. Strawn JR, Moldauer L, Hahn RD, et al. A multicenter double-blind, placebo-controlled trial of escitalopram in children and adolescents with Generalized Anxiety Disorder. J Child Adolesc Psychopharmacol 2023;33(3):91–100.
11. Birmaher B, Axelson DA, Monk K, et al. Fluoxetine for the treatment of childhood anxiety disorders. J Am Acad Child Adolesc Psychiatry 2003;42(4):415–23.

12. Clark DB, Birmaher B, Axelson D, et al. Fluoxetine for the treatment of childhood anxiety disorders: open-label, long-term extension to a controlled trial. J Am Acad Child Adolesc Psychiatry 2005;44(12):1263–70.

13. Beidel DC, Turner SM, Sallee FR, et al. SET-C versus fluoxetine in the treatment of childhood social phobia. Journal of the American Academy of Child & Adolescent Psychiatry 2007;46(12):1622–32.

14. Birmaher B, Waterman GS, Ryan N, et al. Fluoxetine for childhood anxiety disorders. J Am Acad Child Adolesc Psychiatry 1994;33(7):993–9.

15. Fairbanks JM, Pine DS, Tancer NK, et al. Open fluoxetine treatment of mixed anxiety disorders in children and adolescents. *J Child Adolesc Psychopharmacol.* Spring 1997;7(1):17–29.

16. Rynn MA, Siqueland L, Rickels K. Placebo-controlled trial of sertraline in the treatment of children with generalized anxiety disorder. Am J Psychiatry Dec 2001; 158(12):2008–14.

17. Compton SN, Grant PJ, Chrisman AK, et al. Sertraline in children and adolescents with social anxiety disorder: an open trial. J Am Acad Child Adolesc Psychiatry 2001;40(5):564–71.

18. Ginsburg GS, Kendall PC, Sakolsky D, et al. Remission after acute treatment in children and adolescents with anxiety disorders: findings from the CAMS. J Consult Clin Psychol 2011;79(6):806–13.

19. Strawn JR, Mills JA, Suresh V, et al. Combining selective serotonin reuptake inhibitors and cognitive behavioral therapy in youth with depression and anxiety. J Affect Disord 2022;298(Pt A):292–300.

20. Rynn MA, Walkup JT, Compton SN, et al. Child/Adolescent anxiety multimodal study: evaluating safety. J Am Acad Child Adolesc Psychiatry 2015;54(3): 180–90.

21. Piacentini J, Bennett S, Compton SN, et al. 24- and 36-week outcomes for the child/adolescent anxiety multimodal study (CAMS). J Am Acad Child Adolesc Psychiatry 2014;53(3):297–310.

22. Walkup JT, Labellarte MJ, Riddle MA, et al. Fluvoxamine for the treatment of anxiety disorders in children and adolescents. N Engl J Med 2001;344(17):1279–85.

23. Walkup J, Labellarte M, Riddle MA, et al. Treatment of pediatric anxiety disorders: an open-label extension of the research units on pediatric psychopharmacology anxiety study. *J Child Adolesc Psychopharmacol.* Fall 2002;12(3):175–88.

24. Wagner KD, Berard R, Stein MB, et al. A multicenter, randomized, double-blind, placebo-controlled trial of paroxetine in children and adolescents with social anxiety disorder. Arch Gen Psychiatr 2004;61(11):1153–62.

25. Rynn MA, Riddle MA, Yeung PP, et al. Efficacy and safety of extended-release venlafaxine in the treatment of generalized anxiety disorder in children and adolescents: two placebo-controlled trials. Am J Psychiatry 2007;164(2):290–300.

26. March JS, Entusah AR, Rynn M, et al. A randomized controlled trial of venlafaxine ER versus placebo in pediatric social anxiety disorder. Biol Psychiatr 2007; 62(10):1149–54.

27. Strawn JR, Prakash A, Zhang Q, et al. A randomized, placebo-controlled study of duloxetine for the treatment of children and adolescents with generalized anxiety disorder. J Am Acad Child Adolesc Psychiatry 2015;54(4):283–93.

28. Geller D, Donnelly C, Lopez F, et al. Atomoxetine treatment for pediatric patients with attention-deficit/hyperactivity disorder with comorbid anxiety disorder. Journal of the American Academy of Child & Adolescent Psychiatry 2007;46(9): 1119–27.

29. Stimpfl JN, Mills JA, Strawn JR. Pharmacologic predictors of benzodiazepine response trajectory in anxiety disorders: a Bayesian hierarchical modeling meta-analysis. CNS Spectr 2021;1–8.

30. Simeon JG, Ferguson HB. Alprazolam effects in children with anxiety disorders. Can J Psychiatry 1987;32(7):570–4.

31. Simeon JG, Ferguson HB, Knott V, et al. Clinical, cognitive, and neurophysiological effects of alprazolam in children and adolescents with overanxious and avoidant disorders. J Am Acad Child Adolesc Psychiatry 1992;31(1):29–33.

32. Graae F, Milner J, Rizzotto L, et al. Clonazepam in childhood anxiety disorders. Journal of the American Academy of Child & Adolescent Psychiatry 1994; 33(3):372–6.

33. Bernstein GA, Garfinkel BD, Borchardt CM. Comparative studies of pharmacotherapy for school refusal. J Am Acad Child Adolesc Psychiatry 1990;29(5): 773–81.

34. Strawn JR, Mills JA, Cornwall GJ, et al. Buspirone in children and adolescents with anxiety: a review and bayesian analysis of abandoned randomized controlled trials. J Child Adolesc Psychopharmacol 2018;28(1):2–9.

35. Kutcher SP, Reiter S, Gardner DM, et al. The pharmacotherapy of anxiety disorders in children and adolescents. Psychiatr Clin North Am 1992;15(1):41–67.

36. Salazar DE, Frackiewicz EJ, Dockens R, et al. Pharmacokinetics and tolerability of buspirone during oral administration to children and adolescents with anxiety disorder and normal healthy adults. J Clin Pharmacol 2001;41(12):1351–8.

37. Strawn JR, Compton SN, Robertson B, et al. Extended release guanfacine in pediatric anxiety disorders: a pilot, randomized, placebo-controlled trial. J Child Adolesc Psychopharmacol 2017;27(1):29–37.

38. Sallee FR, Lyne A, Wigal T, et al. Long-term safety and efficacy of guanfacine extended release in children and adolescents with attention-deficit/hyperactivity disorder. J Child Adolesc Psychopharmacol 2009;19(3):215–26.

39. Gittelman-Klein R, Klein DF. Controlled imipramine treatment of school phobia. Arch Gen Psychiatr 1971;25(3):204–7.

40. Klein RG, Koplewicz HS, Kanner A. Imipramine treatment of children with separation anxiety disorder. J Am Acad Child Adolesc Psychiatry 1992;31(1):21–8.

41. Bernstein GA, Borchardt CM, Perwien AR, et al. Imipramine plus cognitive-behavioral therapy in the treatment of school refusal. J Am Acad Child Adolesc Psychiatry 2000;39(3):276–83.

42. Kendall PC. Treating anxiety disorders in children: results of a randomized clinical trial. J Consult Clin Psychol 1994;62(1):100–10.

43. Kendall PC, Flannery-Schroeder E, Panichelli-Mindel SM, et al. Therapy for youths with anxiety disorders: a second randomized clinical trial. J Consult Clin Psychol 1997;65(3):366–80.

44. Barrett PM, Dadds MR, Rapee RM. Family treatment of childhood anxiety: a controlled trial. J Consult Clin Psychol 1996;64(2):333.

45. James A, Soler A, Weatherall R. Cognitive behavioural therapy for anxiety disorders in children and adolescents. Cochrane Database Syst Rev 2005;4:1–35.

46. Ginsburg GS, Becker-Haimes EM, Keeton C, et al. Results from the child/adolescent anxiety multimodal extended long-term study (CAMELS): primary anxiety outcomes. Journal of the American Academy of Child & Adolescent Psychiatry 2018;57(7):471–80.

47. Connolly SD, Bernstein GA. Practice parameter for the assessment and treatment of children and adolescents with anxiety disorders. J Am Acad Child Adolesc Psychiatry 2007;46(2):267–83.

48. Strawn JR, Welge JA, Wehry AM, et al. Efficacy and tolerability of antidepressants in pediatric anxiety disorders: a systematic review and meta-analysis. Depress Anxiety 2015;32(3):149–57.
49. Mills JA, Strawn JR. Antidepressant tolerability in pediatric anxiety and obsessive-compulsive disorders: a bayesian hierarchical modeling meta-analysis. J Am Acad Child Adolesc Psychiatry 2020;59(11):1240–51.
50. Strawn JR, Poweleit EA, Ramsey LB. CYP2C19-guided escitalopram and sertraline dosing in pediatric patients: a pharmacokinetic modeling study. J Child Adolesc Psychopharmacol 2019;29(5):340–7.
51. Poweleit E, Vaughn S, Desta Z, et al. CYP2C19 metabolizer status predicts sertraline and escitalopram pharmacokinetics in children and adolescents. Paper presented at: neuropsychopharmacology 2021.
52. Aldrich SL, Poweleit EA, Prows CA, et al. Influence of CYP2C19 metabolizer status on escitalopram/citalopram tolerability and response in youth with anxiety and depressive disorders. Front Pharmacol 2019;99.
53. Genetics ISoP. Genetic Testing and Psychiatric Disorders. A Statement from the International Society of Psychiatric Genetics 2019. Available at: https://ispg.net/genetic-testing-statement/. Accessed March 17, 2023.
54. Ramsey LB, Namerow LB, Bishop JR, et al. Thoughtful clinical use of pharmacogenetics in child and adolescent psychopharmacology. Journal of the American Academy of Child and Adolescent Psychiatry 2021;60(6):660.
55. Strawn JR. 16.1 principles of pharmacogenetic testing in children and adolescents. Journal of the American Academy of Child & Adolescent Psychiatry 2022;61(10):S300–1.

# Neurobiology of Treatment in Pediatric Anxiety Disorders

W. Thomas Baumel, MD[a],*, Jeffrey R. Strawn, MD[a,b,c]

## KEYWORDS

- Anxiety • Neuroimaging • Selective serotonin reuptake inhibitor (SSRI)
- Cognitive behavioral therapy (CBT) • Psychotherapy • Treatment

## KEY POINTS

- APrefrontal and cingulate activity can predict treatment response with either selective serotonin reuptake inhibitors (SSRIs) or psychotherapy. SSRIs and psychotherapies alter activity in similar brain regions that serve as hubs of neuronal synthesis among networks that underlie stimulus-driven attention, error monitoring, task planning, and introspection.
- Individual brain regions work in concert through analog, parallel processing. Thus, treatment-related changes can have ripple effects throughout the multiple circuits.
- We continue to approach a point where baseline neurobiology and neurobiological change can be matched with "outputs" in neuropsychiatric tasks, scales, and symptomology, which may be leveraged to match specific treatments with specific patients who are most likely to robustly respond.

## INTRODUCTION

Anxiety disorders are the sixth leading cause of disability worldwide in those aged 10 to 24 years[1] and affect 7.3% of the global population. They are characterized by alterations in specific brain circuits that subserve fear processing and other psychological processes implicated in the pathogenesis of anxiety disorders. Importantly, while anxiety disorders can be effectively treated with selective serotonin reuptake inhibitors (SSRIs) and psychotherapies, including cognitive behavioral therapy (CBT),[2–6] the way in which these treatments interact with the neurocircuitry of anxiety disorders is poorly understood. In general, treatment-related changes in brain function often

[a] Department of Psychiatry and Behavioral Neuroscience, Anxiety Disorders Research Program, College of Medicine, University of Cincinnati, Box 670559, 260 Stetson Street, Suite 3200, Cincinnati, OH 45267-0559, USA; [b] Division of Child and Adolescent Psychiatry, Department of Pediatrics, Cincinnati Children's Hospital Medical Center, Cincinnati, OH, USA; [c] Division of Clinical Pharmacology, Department of Pediatrics, Cincinnati Children's Hospital Medical Center, Cincinnati, OH, USA
* Corresponding author.
*E-mail address:* baumelwt@mail.uc.edu

Child Adolesc Psychiatric Clin N Am 32 (2023) 589–600
https://doi.org/10.1016/j.chc.2023.02.005
1056-4993/23/© 2023 Elsevier Inc. All rights reserved.

childpsych.theclinics.com

involve the amygdala and prefrontal regions.[7] Understanding how successful treatments engage specific brain circuits in pediatric patients with anxiety disorders could enhance our understanding treatment engagement and identify predictors of treatment response.[8,9]

In youth with anxiety disorders, the amygdala is often overactivated in response to negatively valanced stimuli.[10] Differential activation is also observed during attentional and emotional processing tasks in the anterior cingulate cortex (ACC) and prefrontal cortex (PFC) regions such as the ventrolateral PFC (vlPFC) and dorsomedial PFC (dmPFC).[10,11] Importantly, these regions are important hubs for functional networks including the default mode,[12-14] cingulo-opercular,[15,16] fronto-parietal,[15,16] and ventral attention networks.[17-19] And, dysfunction in each of these networks may disrupt psychological processes leading to symptoms that form the constellation of anxiety disorders.[20,21]

Additionally, compared with healthy youth, children and adolescents with anxiety disorders show alterations in the structural neurobiology. Structural brain studies reveal decreased gray matter volume in the amygdala, precuneus, cuneus, posterior cingulate cortex, and insula.[22-24] When looking at cortical thickness—which is influenced in part by cellular-level developmental processes such as synaptic pruning and cortical neuronal population shifts—the inferior and middle temporal cortices, precentral gyrus, and the ventromedial PFC (vmPFC) have increased thickness in anxious youths.[25,26]

Considered together, these studies indicate that anxiety syndromes change functional activity, structure, and connectivity in the amygdala and other regions that subserve emotion processing, attention, self-reflective thinking, and error monitoring. Normalization of these aberrant changes might mechanistically relate to treatment-specific improvement in anxiety.

Herein, we review how the neurofunctional and neurostructural aspects of pediatric anxiety disorders interact with successful treatment. We review studies of children and adolescents with "triad" anxiety disorders—including generalized, separation, and social anxiety disorders—who are treated with psychotherapy (most commonly CBT) or pharmacotherapy (most commonly SSRIs). We surveyed the literature for neurobiological predictors of treatment efficacy and treatment-related brain changes. These findings may allow the field to move toward precision medicine, selecting particular therapies from the psychiatric armamentarium that best fits the patient's neurobiological phenotype.

In general, few studies have examined predictors of efficacy and treatment-related changes in pediatric anxiety disorders, especially when compared with the extant literature in adults with anxiety or mood disorders. Regarding functional neuroimaging studies, alterations in networks involved in limbic circuitry, executive function, and attention are implicated as predictors of treatment response or treatment-related changes. To date, 2 studies have examined structural predictors of treatment efficacy, and none have examined treatment-related changes in brain structure.

### Functional Neuroimaging Predictors of Treatment Success

Studies of neurofunctional predictors of treatment efficacy in youth with anxiety disorders largely focus on adolescents.[9,27-30] In general, these studies include youth with generalized anxiety disorder (GAD) as well as those with social and separation anxiety disorders, and include psychotherapy and SSRIs.

#### Functional neuroimaging predictors of psychotherapy treatment success
Studies examining baseline brain activation patterns that predict psychotherapeutic response largely focused on CBT with the exception of one study of mindfulness-

based cognitive therapy (MBCT). Additionally, the majority of studies used multiarm approaches in which patients receiv either psychotherapy or anSSRIs with intragroup and intergroup analyses.

In a region of interest approach examining the amygdala, decreased left amygdala activation to emotional faces in 12 adolescents with GAD predicted CBT and fluoxetine-related improvement.[27] In a sequential analysis of 9 adolescents with GAD, whole brain analysis revealed MBCT-related changes in the left ACC and right anterior insula. Using these 2 regions as regions of interest, increased baseline activation to emotional images in both regions predicted improvement in anxiety symptoms following MBCT.[28] In a mixed diagnostic sample of 121 adolescents (56% GAD, 44% social anxiety disorder), region of interest analysis of the dorsal ACC (dACC) and dmPFC revealed decreased baseline response to implicit threat processing predicted greater anxiety symptom improvement following either CBT or sertraline monotherapy with no influence shown for either treatment type or primary diagnosis.[30] Using a whole brain analysis of adolescents treated with CBT or sertraline, baseline increased activity to threatening faces in the dorsolateral PFC (dlPFC), vlPFC, precentral gyrus, and postcentral gyrus predicted greater improvement in anxiety symptoms following treatment.[29] Pretreatment Pediatric Anxiety Rating Scale (PARS) was included as a covariate.

### Functional neuroimaging predictors of selective serotonin reuptake inhibitor treatment response

Neurofunctional studies of SSRI-treated pediatric patients with anxiety disorders largely focus on the amygdala given its central importance within limbic fear circuits. In the first study, Maslowsky examined 14 youth with GAD and found that fluoxetine treatment increased activation within the vlPFC.[31] In a subsequent study of adolescents with GAD, those with less amygdala activation to emotional faces before treatment had greater improvement with CBT and fluoxetine.[27] Additionally, in a large study of adolescents with mixed anxiety disorders (N= 121, 56% with GAD and 44% social anxiety disorder), decreased activation of the dACC and dmPFC before treatment predicted greater improvement with both CBT and sertraline regardless of the patient's primary diagnosis.[30] Finally, using a whole brain analysis in these CBT or sertraline-treated adolescents activity in the dlPFC, vlPFC, precentral gyrus, and postcentral gyrus before treatment predicted greater improvement.[29]

Using a resting-state functional connectivity MRI (rs-fcMRI) analysis, the first 2 weeks of treatment with escitalopram—but not placebo—increased amygdala-vlPFC connectivity in adolescents with GAD (**Fig. 1**). Further, in escitalopram-treated (but not placebo-treated) patients, the magnitude of increases in amygdala-vlPFC, particularly the basolateral amygdala–vlPFC, functional connectivity, predicted the trajectory of anxiety symptom reduction during 8 weeks. Indeed, it did so better than baseline amygdala functional connectivity and demographic characteristics.[9] Interestingly, the strength of the connectivity changes originated in the basolateral amygdala (see **Fig. 1**), which is the region of the amygdala that receives information about the external environment from the sensory thalamus and neocortices, and reciprocally projects to cortical regions implicated in the pathophysiology of anxiety disorders.[32] Additionally, within the basolateral amygdala, serotonin (5-HT) regulates neuronal responses to aversive sensory cues.[33,34]

### Structural Predictors of Treatment Response in Pediatric Anxiety Disorders

Neurostructural aspects of pediatric anxiety disorders are frequently probed by measuring gray matter volume and cortical thickness while white matter integrity

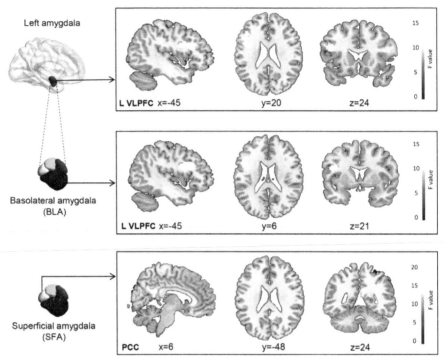

**Fig. 1.** Treatment-by-time interaction in amygdala- and amygdala subdivision–based functional connectivity (FC) in adolescents with generalized anxiety disorder. BLA, basolateral amygdala; L, left; PCC, posterior cingulate cortex; SFA, superficial amygdala; VLPFC, ventrolateral prefrontal cortex. *P < .05; **P < .001. (*Reprinted from* JAACAP, 60(10), Lu Lu, Jeffrey A. Mills, Hailong Li, Heidi K. Schroeder, Sarah A. Mossman, Sara T. Varney, Kim M. Cecil, Xiaoqi Huang, Qiyong Gong, Laura B. Ramsey, Melissa P. DelBello, John A. Sweeney, Jeffrey R. Strawn, Acute Neurofunctional Effects of Escitalopram in Pediatric Anxiety: A Double-Blind, Placebo-Controlled Trial, 1309-88, 2021, with permission from Elsevier.)

and structure are often evaluated with diffusion-tensor imaging (DTI). These approaches are helpful in describing how the brains of individuals with anxiety disorders may structurally differ from those without anxiety and can help to link structure and function. Moreover, they may point toward aberrant "hardwiring," which may predispose to a greater or lesser "software" (ie, functional activity) response to treatment.

Neurostructural studies of treatment-related changes can provide insight to how treatments may change brain activity and connectivity, and from inferring how structure may affect function. These neurostructural analyses may be limited, however, in that most studies occur over the time course of weeks to months, which may be inadequate to capture underlying neurostructural changes. At the neuronal unit, structural changes (eg, lower synaptic density) have been observed in lower animals as result of serotonergic insufficiency.[35] Additionally, in mice, SSRIs have also been linked to increasing brain-derived neurotrophic factor, a key factor for long-term potentiation and neuroplasticity.[36,37]

Studying the structural predictors of treatment response in pediatric anxiety disorders, Gold and colleagues examined structural correlates to anxiety severity and treatment response in 75 youths with an anxiety diagnosis. Worse outcomes were associated with decreased cortical thickness in the parietal and occipital cortices at baseline despite not being associated with baseline anxiety.[25] Burkhouse and colleagues[38] also examined structural predictors of treatment efficacy. In children with anxiety disorders (N = 55), greater left nucleus accumbens volume predicted greater improvement in anxiety symptoms following 12 weeks of treatment with either CBT or sertraline. Contrary to their hypothesis, there was no evidence that baseline vmPFC or amygdala volume predicted treatment efficacy following 12 weeks of treatment with either CBT or sertraline.[38] These findings are intriguing given neurobiological studies have often observed decreased gray matter volume in the amygdalas of children and adolescents with anxiety disorders, when compared with nonanxious peers.[22–24] This may suggest that the "hardwiring" of key limbic hubs may not predict treatment efficacy. Rather, the degree to which the aberrant hardwiring affects the functional capabilities may be the critical factor in predicting efficacy. Moreover, perhaps, faciliatory regions such as the nucleus accumbens, are "upregulated" in volume to make up for a hyperfunctional limbic fear circuit and the degree to which these faciliatory regions are upregulated may predict increased likelihood to improve.

### Treatment Effects on Functional Neuroimaging

A half dozen trials have examined the functional neurophysiologic changes following treatment in youth with anxiety disorders. In general, these studies are small (range 9–25 patients with the exception of a larger electroencephalogram [EEG] study) and use the PARS[39] to measure change in anxiety severity. The functional neuroimaging tasks vary across studies and innclude rs-fcMRI, dot-probe tasks, viewing emotional faces, Eriksen flanker task, and a continuous processing task with emotional and neutral distractors.

#### Psychotherapy effects on functional neuroimaging

Four studies examined neurofunctional changes after psychotherapeutic treatment. Psychotherapeutic approaches include largely cognitive approaches ($n_{CBT} = 4$, $n_{MBCT} = 1$) with one using a form of supportive psychotherapy. They largely implicate regions in the lateral PFC and ACC as regions affected by treatment.

Using a region of interest approach encompassing the right vlPFC and bilateral amygdala, CBT or fluoxetine monotherapy increased vlPFC activation in response to angry faces during the dot probe task in adolescents with GAD.[31]

We used whole brain analysis of a continuous processing task with emotional and neutral distractors task in adolescents with GAD (some with comorbid social and/or separation anxiety disorder) to examine the neurofunctional effects of MBCT in anxious youths. In this sample, we observed enhanced activation of the lentiform nucleus, thalamus, bilateral insula, and left ACC in response to emotional stimuli.[28] Burkhouse and colleagues examined CBT-related (and sertraline-related) effects in adolescents with GAD (N = 25) using whole brain analysis of an emotional face viewing paradigm. Rostral ACC activity in response to emotional faces increased following treatment compared with a healthy control group.[40]

Error-related negativity is a negative EEG deflection that occurs about 100 milliseconds after an inaccuracy and is a marker of an overactive error monitoring system.[41] In a study of 100 youth with an anxiety disorders (*Diagnostic and Statistical Manual-IV* [DSM-IV] criteria), EEG demonstrated an increased error-related negativity compared with healthy controls (N = 30) at baseline.[42] After 16 sessions of CBT or a form of supportive psychotherapy called child-centered therapy, there was no change in the magnitude of the error-related negativity although anxiety symptoms improved in both groups.[42]

*Selective serotonin reuptake inhibitor effects on functional neuroimaging*

Four studies have examined neurofunctional changes after pharmacologic treatment and these studies all involved SSRIs ($n_{sertraline} = 1$, $n_{fluoxetine} = 2$, and $n_{escitalopram} = 2$). Here, as well, regions in the lateral PFC and ACC were observed to change functional activation patterns following treatment suggesting neurobiologic overlap in the substrates of psychotherapeutic and pharmacologic treatment.

As described above, using the right vlPFC and bilateral amygdala as regions of interest during a dot probe task, CBT, or fluoxetine monotherapy for adolescents with GAD increased right vlPFC activation in response to angry faces.[31]

Using whole brain analyses as previously described, Burkhouse and colleagues examined sertraline-related (and CBT-related) effects in adolescents with various anxiety disorders (GAD, social anxiety, and separation anxiety disorders). Following treatment, rostral ACC activity increased in response to emotional faces compared with a healthy control group.[40]

Two studies examined treatment-related changes in functional connectivity in adolescents with GAD randomized to escitalopram or placebo. In one, rs-fcMRI was acquired before and after 2 weeks of treatment. During the first 2 weeks of treatment, escitalopram—but not placebo—increased amygdala-vlPFC connectivity. Additionally, this early, 2-week functional connectivity change predicted symptom improvement over the subsequent 6 weeks of treatment in youth who received escitalopram but not in those who received placebo.[43] A second study examined adolescents with GAD (N = 36) randomized to 8 weeks of placebo or escitalopram.[8] During emotional processing, adolescents treated with escitalopram, compared with placebo, exhibited more negative right amygdala to bilateral vmPFC connectivity and more positive left amygdala to right angular gyrus connectivity.[8]

## SUMMARY

Herein, we have reviewed the current literature on the neurobiological predictors of treatment efficacy and the treatment-related changes in neurobiology. The existing literature is best viewed as a partially constructed scaffold.[7] Heterogeneity in population, task, neuroimaging modality, and analytic approach preclude more traditional, robust syntheses such as meta-analysis. However, it serves as a strong foundation to construct a vigorous, harmonized understanding of biomarkers in pediatric anxiety syndromes.

Both pharmacologic and psychotherapeutic treatment-related changes increase activity in structures implicated in prefrontal regulatory circuits such as the vlPFC, insula, and ACC (**Fig. 2**).[28,31,40] Additionally, the functional connectivity of these regions with the amygdala is enhanced following pharmacological treatment.[8,43] This suggests overlapping neurocircuit-level mechanisms of action across therapeutic modalities; treatment enhances regulatory circuits and allows for more effective attenuation of overactive limbic signals.

A surfeit of brain regions have been identified as potential biomarkers of treatment in anxiety disorders. Each, in isolation, can be viewed in a reductionistic fashion to represent a brain region's altered response during attention, emotional processing, error monitoring, and so forth. Studying brain regions in isolation can prove fruitful by revealing insights into individual pathways. However, such a narrow perspective neglects the enriched context of the inter-network synthesis and parallel integration inherent to the brain. For example, disruptions in a regions implicated in attention may have ripple effects that affect error monitoring and vice versa.

It is crucial to keep in mind that these brain regions act in concert in functional networks. These networks, themselves, are interconnected and cross modulating, with

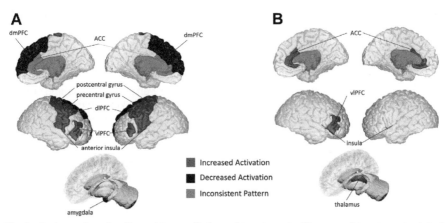

**Fig. 2.** Brain regions implicated in prediction of treatment efficacy and treatment-related change. (*A*) Brain regions observed to predict treatment efficacy with pharmacotherapy and/or psychotherapy. (*B*) Brain regions detected in treatment-related change with pharmacotherapy and/or psychotherapy. (Drawings generated using BrainPainter. A software for the visualization of brain structures. Marinescu, Razvan, Eshaghi, Arman, Alexander, Daniel, & Golland, Polina. 2019.)

each level of complexity endowing new properties to the system. When examining the extant literature, regions that serve as key hubs in the default mode network (eg, ACC, mPFC), ventral attention network (eg, vlPFC), cingulo-opercular/salience network (eg, ACC, anterior insula, thalamus), and fronto-parietal/executive control network (eg, dlPFC, middle cingulate gyrus) have been identified as preliminarily biomarkers of treatment success and neurobiological change.

We are just beginning to understand the complex interconnections of the human mind through coordinated, multisite investigational undertaking such as the Human Connectome Project.[44,45] By understanding the complicated internetwork workings of the brain, we may conduct "lesion network mapping" in different psychopathologies and neuropsychiatric symptoms to uncover new treatment targets.[46]

Perturbations in specific circuits in anxiety syndromes, and how they manifest phenomenologically in patients, have been hypothesized.[20,21] Building on these earlier hypotheses, recent research has uncovered altered intranetwork and internetwork connectivities in pediatric anxiety disorders and associated these functional brain changes with anxiety disorder experiences.

In a pediatric sample, higher levels of anxiety was associated with altered connectivity between the cingulo-opercular network and the ventral attention, default mode, and visual networks. In particular, the altered connectivity between the ventral attention and cingulo-opercular networks was related to higher clinician-rated anxiety and more intense stimulus-driven attention.[47]

Moreover, internetwork connectivity may be modified by the psychiatric armamentarium. In a recent double-blind, placebo-controlled trial (reviewed above), escitalopram was associated with more negative right amygdala to bilateral vmPFC and greater positive left amygdala to right angular gyrus connectivity. Greater magnitude of these connectivity changes at 2 weeks predicted greater improvement in anxiety symptoms at 8 weeks.[8] This suggests that treatment with SSRI may modulate the internetwork communication between hubs of the limbic fear circuitry (ie, the amygdala) with the default mode network (ie, vmPFC) and salience, ventral attention, and executive control networks (ie, angular gyrus region). This may lead to decreased fear modulation regarding self-referential observation, attentional control, and executive function.

## CLINICAL GUIDANCE

At this point, the science is neither advanced enough to warrant neuroimaging studies of patients to parse patients into "Likely Responder" or "Likely Under-responder" buckets nor to monitor clinical effect. Nevertheless, we can increasingly appreciate internetwork connectivity "lesions" in anxious syndromes, how they relate to measurable psychological processes, and how pharmacotherapies and psychotherapies differentially modify neurofunctional communications implicated in these processes. With these appreciations, we may leverage "fingerprints" in neuroimaging with "outputs" in neuropsychiatric tasks, scales, and experience to match specific treatments with specific patients.[48,49] For example, someone with anxious, ruminating self-referential thought may benefit from escitalopram with its modulation of limbic-default mode network connectivity.

Such leveraging of neuroimaging fingerprints to neuropsychiatric outputs may help address the heterogeneity in treatment response. Up to 40% of patients fail to significantly improve following first-line intervention.[2] This may be, in part, due to meaningfully different patterns of neurobiological diversity that exist in anxiety disorders. The current pediatric anxiety literature may reflect this with its current surfeit of neurobiological biomarkers across studies with different populations. Indeed, recently, 3 functional subdivisions within the amygdala have been proposed based on independently replicated data. These subdivisions are correlated preferentially with the default mode network, dorsal attention, and fronto-parietal networks, and nonpreferentially, respectively. Critically, in this population, there was substantial across-subject variation in the distribution and magnitude of amygdala functional connectivity with the cerebral cortex.[50] We can move beyond the current one-size-fits-all selection of psychiatric interventions, toward more nuanced therapeutic strategies that recognize the important role of individual neuronal differences.

Further, trials such as the Sequenced Treatment Alternatives to Relieve Depression (STAR*D) Study indicate that an adequate trial of an SSRI is 6 to 8 weeks.[51] Critically, there should be observed improvements in symptomatology in the first few weeks. The importance of early symptom improvement was shown in a recent study of anxious depression treated with escitalopram.[52] Early 2-week improvement in anxiety symptoms was positively predictive of response or remission of anxious (and depressive) symptoms at 8 weeks. Moreover, the lack of improvement in anxiety symptoms at 2 weeks of SSRI treatment was predictive of nonresponse and nonremission once an adequate trial was reached at 8 weeks.[52] These results are interesting in light of data from our recent randomized, placebo-controlled trial of escitalopram. As reviewed, the magnitude of functional connectivity change between the basolateral amygdala and vmPFC at 2-weeks of treatment with escitalopram—and not baseline functional connectivity—predicted treatment efficacy at 8 weeks.[8]

Considered together, these findings, urge greater attention to short-term changes in symptom severity and functional neurobiology as a way of anticipating the treatment trajectory of our patients. For example, we may be able to leverage short-term data at 2 weeks, such as no symptom improvement or no change in functional connectivity, as evidence to switch treatment tracks or more quickly titrate a tolerated medication earlier than the 8 weeks of an adequate trial. In this way, an ultimately ineffective treatment (ie, one that leads to no response or remission) may be discontinued earlier and the patient transitioned to a second medication of the same or different class. Quicker transition to an ultimately effective medication and dosage may reduce morbidity and neurologic "kindling." Through more sophisticated approaches such as these, we can leverage the likelihood of normalizing a patient's specific pattern of activation or connectivity, which may prove more fruitful for our patients.

## CLINICS CARE POINTS

- Early change in neurobiology may reflect early symptom improvement and may predict clinical improvement
- Neurobiologic treatment-related changes may be reflected in symptom ratings. Understanding this relationship will be fundamental to translational work
- Reproducible, large clinical trials are needed to translate neuroimaging data into clinically actionable interventions and approaches

## DECLARATION OF INTERESTS

Dr Strawn has received research support from the Yung Family Foundation, the National Institutes of Health (NIMH/NIEHS), United States, the National Center for Advancing Translational Sciences, the Patient Centered Outcomes Research Institute (PCORI) and Abbvie. He has received material support from Myriad Health and royalties from 3 texts (Springer). Dr Strawn serves as an author for *UpToDate* and an Associate Editor for *Current Psychiatry* and has provided consultation to the FDA, Cereval and IntraCellular Therapeutics. Views expressed within this article represent those of the authors and are not intended to represent the position of NIMH, United States, the National Institutes of Health (NIH), United States, or the Department of Health and Human Services.

## ACKNOWLEDGMENTS

This work was supported by the Yung Family Foundation and the Eunice Kennedy Shriver National Institute of Child Health and Human Development (NICHD, R01HD099775 [JRS] and R01HD098757 [JRS]).

## REFERENCES

1. Abbafati C, Machado DB, Cislaghi B, et al. Global burden of 369 diseases and injuries in 204 countries and territories, 1990–2019: a systematic analysis for the Global Burden of Disease Study 2019. Lancet 2020;396(10258):1204–22.
2. Walkup JT, Albano AM, Piacentini J, et al. Cognitive behavioral therapy, sertraline, or a combination in childhood anxiety. N Engl J Med 2008;359(26):2753–66.
3. Jakubovski E, Johnson JA, Nasir M, et al. Systematic review and meta-analysis: dose-response curve of SSRIs and SNRIs in anxiety disorders. Depress Anxiety 2019;36(3):198–212.
4. Wang Z, Whiteside SP, Sim L, et al. Comparative effectiveness and safety of cognitive behavioral therapy and pharmacotherapy for childhood anxiety disorders: a systematic review and meta-analysis. JAMA Pediatr 2017;171(11):1049–56.
5. Locher C, Koechlin H, Zion SR, et al. Efficacy and safety of selective serotonin reuptake inhibitors, serotonin-norepinephrine reuptake inhibitors, and placebo

for common psychiatric disorders among children and adolescents: a systematic review and meta-analysis. JAMA Psychiatry 2017;74(10):1011–20.

6. Strawn JR, Welge JA, Wehry AM, et al. Efficacy and tolerability of antidepressants in pediatric anxiety disorders: a systematic review and meta-analysis. Depress Anxiety 2015;32(3):149–1157.

7. Baumel WT, Lu L, Huang X, et al. Neurocircuitry of treatment in anxiety disorders. Biomarkers in Neuropsychiatry 2022;6:100052.

8. Lu L, Li H, Baumel WT, et al. Acute neurofunctional effects of escitalopram during emotional processing in pediatric anxiety: a double-blind, placebo-controlled trial. Neuropsychopharmacology 2021. https://doi.org/10.1038/s41386-021-01186-0.

9. Lu L, Mills JA, Li H, et al. Acute Neurofunctional effects of escitalopram in pediatric anxiety: a double-blind, placebo-controlled trial. J Am Acad Child Adolesc Psychiatry 2021;60(10):1309–18.

10. Blackford JU, Pine DS. Neural substrates of childhood anxiety disorders a review of neuroimaging findings. Child Adolesc Psychiatr Clin N Am 2012;21(3):501–25.

11. Strawn JR, Lu L, Peris TS, et al. Research review: pediatric anxiety disorders – what have we learnt in the last 10 years? J Child Psychol Psychiatry Allied Discip 2021;62(2):114–39.

12. Raichle ME, MacLeod AM, Snyder AZ, et al. A default mode of brain function. Proc Natl Acad Sci U S A 2001;98(2):676–82.

13. Greicius MD, Krasnow B, Reiss AL, et al. Functional connectivity in the resting brain: a network analysis of the default mode hypothesis. Proc Natl Acad Sci U S A 2003;100(1):253–8.

14. Shulman GL, Fiez JA, Corbetta M, et al. Common blood flow changes across visual tasks: II. Decreases in cerebral cortex. J Cogn Neurosci 1997;9(5):648–63.

15. Seeley WW, Menon V, Schatzberg AF, et al. Dissociable intrinsic connectivity networks for salience processing and executive control. J Neurosci 2007;27(9):2349–56.

16. Dosenbach NUF, Fair DA, Cohen AL, et al. A dual-networks architecture of top-down control. Trends Cogn Sci 2008;12(3):99–105.

17. Corbetta M, Patel G, Shulman GL. The reorienting system of the human brain: from environment to theory of mind. Neuron 2008;58(3):306–24.

18. Corbetta M, Shulman GL. Control of goal-directed and stimulus-driven attention in the brain. Nat Rev Neurosci 2002;3(3):201–15.

19. Fox MD, Corbetta M, Snyder AZ, et al. Spontaneous neuronal activity distinguishes human dorsal and ventral attention systems. Proc Natl Acad Sci U S A 2006;103(26):10046–51.

20. Sylvester CM, Corbetta M, Raichle ME, et al. Functional network dysfunction in anxiety and anxiety disorders. Trends Neurosci 2012;35(9):527–35.

21. Williams LM. Precision psychiatry: a neural circuit taxonomy for depression and anxiety. Lancet Psychiatry 2016;3(5):472–80.

22. Milham MP, Nugent AC, Drevets WC, et al. Selective reduction in amygdala volume in pediatric anxiety disorders: a voxel-based morphometry investigation. Biol Psychiatry 2005;57(9):961–6.

23. Mueller SC, Aouidad A, Gorodetsky E, et al. Grey matter volume in adolescent anxiety: an impact of the brain-derived neurotropic factor Val66Met polymorphism? J Am Acad Child Adolesc Psychiatry 2013;52(2):184–95.

24. Strawn JR, Wehry AM, Chu W-J, et al. Neuroanatomic abnormalities in adolescents with generalized anxiety disorder: a voxel-based morphometry study. Depress Anxiety 2013;30(9):2013.

25. Gold AL, Steuber ER, White LK, et al. Cortical thickness and subcortical gray matter volume in pediatric anxiety disorders. Neuropsychopharmacology 2017; 42(12):2423–33.

26. Strawn JR, John Wegman C, Dominick KC, et al. Cortical surface anatomy in pediatric patients with generalized anxiety disorder. J Anxiety Disord 2014;28(7): 717–23.

27. McClure EB, Adler A, Monk CS, et al. fMRI predictors of treatment outcome in pediatric anxiety disorders. Psychopharmacology (Berl) 2007;191(1):97–105.

28. Strawn JR, Cotton S, Luberto CM, et al. Neural function before and after mindfulness-based cognitive therapy in anxious adolescents at risk for developing bipolar disorder. J Child Adolesc Psychopharmacol 2016;26(4):372–9.

29. Kujawa A, Swain JE, Hanna GL, et al. Prefrontal reactivity to social signals of threat as a predictor of treatment response in anxious youth. Neuropsychopharmacology 2016;41(8):1983–90.

30. Burkhouse KL, Kujawa A, Klumpp H, et al. Neural correlates of explicit and implicit emotion processing in relation to treatment response in pediatric anxiety. J Child Psychol Psychiatry Allied Discip 2017;58(5):546–54.

31. Maslowsky J, Mogg K, Bradley BP, et al. A preliminary investigation of neural correlates of treatment in adolescents with generalized anxiety disorder. J Child Adolesc Psychopharmacol 2010;20(2):105–11.

32. Janak PH, Tye KM. From circuits to behaviour in the amygdala. Nature 2015; 517(7534):284–92.

33. Guo JD, O'Flaherty BM, Rainnie DG. Serotonin gating of cortical and thalamic glutamate inputs onto principal neurons of the basolateral amygdala. Neuropharmacology 2017;126:224–32.

34. Bocchio M, McHugh SB, Bannerman DM, et al. Serotonin, amygdala and fear: assembling the puzzle. Front Neural Circuits 2016;10(APR):1–15.

35. Mazer C, Muneyyirci J, Taheny K, et al. Serotonin depletion during synaptogenesis leads to decreased synaptic density and learning deficits in the adult rat: a possible model of neurodevelopmental disorders with cognitive deficits. Brain Res 1997;760(1–2):68–73.

36. Bath KG, Jing DQ, Dincheva I, et al. BDNF Val66Met impairs fluoxetine-induced enhancement of adult hippocampus plasticity. Neuropsychopharmacology 2012; 37(5):1297–304.

37. Duman RS, Aghajanian GK. Synaptic dysfunction in depression: potential therapeutic targets. Science (80) 2012;338(6103):68–72.

38. Burkhouse KL, Jimmy J, Defelice N, et al. Nucleus accumbens volume as a predictor of anxiety symptom improvement following CBT and SSRI treatment in two independent samples. Neuropsychopharmacology 2020;45(3):561–9.

39. The pediatric anxiety rating scale (PARS): development and psychometric properties. J Am Acad Child Adolesc Psychiatry 2002;41(9):1061–9.

40. Burkhouse KL, Kujawa A, Hosseini B, et al. Anterior cingulate activation to implicit threat before and after treatment for pediatric anxiety disorders. Prog Neuro-Psychopharmacol Biol Psychiatry 2018;84:250–6.

41. Gehring WJ, Goss B, Coles MGH, et al. A neural system for error detection and compensation. Psychol Sci 1993;4(6):385–90.

42. Ladouceur CD, Tan PZ, Sharma V, et al. Error-related brain activity in pediatric anxiety disorders remains elevated following individual therapy: a randomized clinical trial. J Child Psychol Psychiatry 2018;59(11):1152–61.

43. Lu L, Mills JA, Li H, et al. Acute neurofunctional effects of escitalopram in pediatric anxiety: a double-blind,placebo-controlled trial. J Am Acad Child Adolesc Psychiatry 2021. https://doi.org/10.1016/j.jaac.2020.11.023.

44. Smith SM, Beckmann CF, Andersson J, et al. Resting-state fMRI in the human connectome project. Neuroimage 2013;80:144–68.

45. Van Essen DC, Smith SM, Barch DM, et al. The Wu-minn human connectome project: an overview. Neuroimage 2013;80:62–79.

46. Fox MD. Mapping symptoms to brain networks with the human connectome. N Engl J Med 2018;379(23):2237–45.

47. Perino MT, Myers MJ, Wheelock MD, et al. Whole-brain resting-state functional connectivity patterns associated with pediatric anxiety and involuntary attention capture. Biol Psychiatry Glob Open Sci 2021;1(3):229–38.

48. Stancil SL, Tumberger J, Strawn JR. Target to treatment: a charge to develop biomarkers of response and tolerability in child and adolescent psychiatry. Clin Transl Sci 2021;(December 2021):816–23. https://doi.org/10.1111/cts.13216.

49. Baumel WT, Mills JA, Schroeder HK, et al. Executive functioning in pediatric anxiety and its relationship to selective serotonin reuptake inhibitor treatment response: a double-blind, placebo-controlled trial. J Child Adolesc Psychopharmacol 2022;32(4):215–23.

50. Sylvester CM, Yu Q, Srivastava BA, et al. Individual-specific functional connectivity of the amygdala: a substrate for precision psychiatry. Proc Natl Acad Sci U S A 2020;117(7):3808–18.

51. Sinyor M, Schaffer A, Levitt A. The sequenced treatment alternatives to relieve depression (STAR*D) trial: a review. Can J Psychiatry 2010;55(3):126–35.

52. Khoo Y, Demchenko I, Frey BN, et al. Baseline anxiety, and early anxiety/depression improvement in anxious depression predicts treatment outcomes with escitalopram: a CAN-BIND-1 study report. J Affect Disord 2022;300(December 2021):50–8.

# Treatment for Anxiety Disorders in the Pediatric Primary Care Setting

Jennifer B. Blossom, PhD[a],*, Nathaniel Jungbluth, PhD[b],
Erin Dillon-Naftolin, MD[b,c,d], William French, MD[b,c,d]

## KEYWORDS

- Integrated care • Pediatric primary care • Anxiety • Cognitive-behavioral therapy
- Pharmacotherapy

## KEY POINTS

- Pediatric anxiety can be effectively managed in integrated pediatric primary care.
- Exposure-based cognitive behavioral therapy is the first-line behavioral intervention for youth anxiety.
- Pharmacotherapy can be effective as a stand-alone treatment or in conjunction with cognitive behavioral therapy.

## BACKGROUND

Anxiety disorders are among the most commonly diagnosed mental health problems in children and adolescents.[1] Without intervention, anxiety disorders in youth are chronic, debilitating, and amplify risk of early morbidity and mortality, such as depression and suicide.[1,2] Unfortunately, youth anxiety rates continue to increase[3] with historic rates due to COVID-19.[4] Primary care is often a more accessible setting for youth and reduces barriers to care such as stigma,[5] and most of the youth are seen by their pediatrician at least annually.[6,7] In many cases, pediatricians are the first clinicians that families approach about mental health concerns and youth with anxiety present to primary care frequently (eg, due to somatic complaints associated with anxiety symptoms).[8-10] Integrated pediatric primary care (IPC), the provision of behavioral health services in primary care settings, increases treatment access and engagement for youth. For youth with anxiety, IPC reduces symptoms and improves functioning.[11,12]

a Department of Psychology, University of Maine, 376 Williams Hall, Orono, ME 04473, USA;
b Seattle Children's, Partnership Access Line, P.O. Box 51023, Seattle, WA 98115-1023, USA;
c Seattle Children's, Child and Adolescent Psychiatry and Behavioral Medicine, M/S OA.5.154, PO Box 5371, Seattle, WA 98145-5005, USA; d University of Washington, Child and Adolescent Psychiatry, Seattle, WA, USA
* Corresponding author.
E-mail address: jennifer.blossom@maine.edu

Child Adolesc Psychiatric Clin N Am 32 (2023) 601–611
https://doi.org/10.1016/j.chc.2023.02.003
1056-4993/23/© 2023 Elsevier Inc. All rights reserved.

## ASSESSMENT, EVALUATION, AND TRIAGE

Consistent with recent United States Preventive Services Task Force (USPSTF) recommendations,[13] universal screening for youth anxiety helps early identification of youth who may benefit from primary care-based intervention. Brief and validated screening measures are ideal for such purposes and useful for measurement-based care. The PROMIS Anxiety Short Form[14] is a brief, validated measure that assesses anxiety for youth as young as 5 years, includes both caregiver and youth forms, and was initially developed for use in integrated care settings. When elevated anxiety is identified, the initial intervention should incorporate psychoeducation about anxiety and introduce treatment options (outlined below). Importantly, when youth are referred to community-based mental health services from the primary care setting, a minority of youth ever initiate services (~30%).[15,16] Now, more than ever, anxiety treatment in IPC is needed. Below, the authors outline a few approaches to anxiety treatment in primary care.

## DISCUSSION

*Behavioral interventions for youth anxiety in primary care*: Evidence-based psychological interventions for pediatric anxiety, namely exposure-based cognitive behavioral therapy,[17,18] improve outcomes for youth, including reducing anxiety-related impairment and delivering secondary prevention of long-term consequences, including suicidality.[19–21] Exposure-based treatment (described in more detail below) involves patients taking steps to face their feared experiences (ie, reducing impairing avoidance; **Box 1**). Despite these promising outcomes, as few as 17.8% of youth ever receive treatment for anxiety, and those who ultimately receive care wait years between problem onset and initiation of treatment.[22] Even fewer youth participate in evidence-based interventions (EBI) for anxiety, thereby increasing both the personal and societal cost of unresolved anxiety.

Cognitive behavioral intervention in primary care is feasible and can be effective. Prior research has supported CBT delivery by nurses,[23] pediatricians,[24] and integrated behavioral health providers (BHPs).[12] Unfortunately, the few studies that have evaluated CBT in IPC have found that exposure is used infrequently, with other, less efficacious approaches (eg, relaxation) taking precedence. Ideally, anxiety intervention in IPC should follow a stepped care approach: providing (1) psychoeducation and family-facing resources about anxiety, (2) brief exposure-based treatment in the primary care setting, and (3) community referral when needed.

Brief exposure-based anxiety treatment can be readily implemented into primary care. Consistent with best practices, the behavioral approaches should prioritize starting exposures as soon as possible (ideally within the first few sessions).[25] After providing initial psychoeducation, clinicians should work with the youth and family to identify primary areas of impairment and collaboratively develop a plan for structured exposures. Effective exposures use an inhibitory learning (IL) approach that effectively and efficiently supports new learning to counteracts previously learned fear responses.[26] IL exposures aim to teach the patient through experiential learning that their fear expectations (that bad things are likely to happen, would be very bad, and could not be coped with) do not match reality so that previously avoided situations are experienced as safe and manageable, and as a result, the body stops producing such a strong, unnecessary fear response.[26] Exposures should be constructed specifically to test out and disconfirm the patient's expectations for unnecessarily avoided situations, which bad outcomes are likely, would be very bad, and the patient would be unable to cope. A hypothetical case example implementing exposure-based treatment is detailed below.

---

**Box 1**
**Overview of exposures**

- Exposure, or brave practice, involves taking steps to face feared situations.

- Exposure is indicated when patients experience significant anxiety in the absence of an objective threat or when patients experience an exaggerated fear response to typical risk situations.

- Key elements of effective exposure include:
  o Ensure that patients understand the rationale for exposure and the exposures are voluntary
  o Identify a feared situation to practice:
    - Consider prioritizing situations for which avoidance is most impairing or disruptive
    - Consider identifying a range of related situations and begin with one that is not too difficult

  o Work with the patient to identify their fear expectations for the situation that are driving their anxious response.
    - Typically, fear expectations outcomes include (1) A bad outcome is very likely, (2) the outcome would be very bad, and (3) the patient will be unable to cope with the outcome.
    - Get specific about patient predictions. For example, the expectation is that if I stay for 5 minutes people will laugh at me and there is an 85% chance of that happening.

  o Identify and prevent any safety behaviors (eg, checking reflection, having a phone or person present) that might interfere with new learning

  o Encourage your patient to stay present in the situation and to notice any body sensations of anxiety to maximize learning

  o Ask your patient questions during and after the exposure to draw attention to new learning
    - What surprised you?
    - How did this match what you expected?

  o Practice repeating the exposure in new contexts

  o Practice incorporating multiple fear cues in one exposure

---

In some cases, youth present with elevated anxiety about situations that involve real stressors, in which case an exposure-based treatment would be contraindicated (eg, anxiety about a class that prompts studying). Before initiating exposure, clinicians should evaluate which treatment approach may be the most effective based on their patient's needs (**Fig. 1**). Below the authors outline specific considerations for a stepped treatment approach (see **Box 2**).

*Step One: Psychoeducation and self-guided resources:* When concerning anxiety has been identified during a primary care visit, the primary care physician (PCP) or other primary care staff can give brief information about anxiety and provide families with self-guided resources that cover the key points of what anxiety is when it is a problem, and strategies to overcome it, including exposure. At that point, families may opt to initiate brave practice independently, or PCPs can refer families to brief exposure-based IPC treatment.

*Step Two: Brief integrated pediatric primary care treatment:* Exposure-based, brief primary care treatment should start with an initial assessment to identify key areas of anxiety-related impairment and rule out other mental health concerns that may impact treatment. Specific comorbid concerns that warrant treatment priority and may require specific attention before initiating anxiety treatment include (but may not be limited to) suicidality or self-harm, trauma, significant mood concerns, or significant behavioral or attentional concerns. If, after initial assessment, anxiety seems to be the primary concern and in the absence of other pressing treatment targets (eg., safety), the

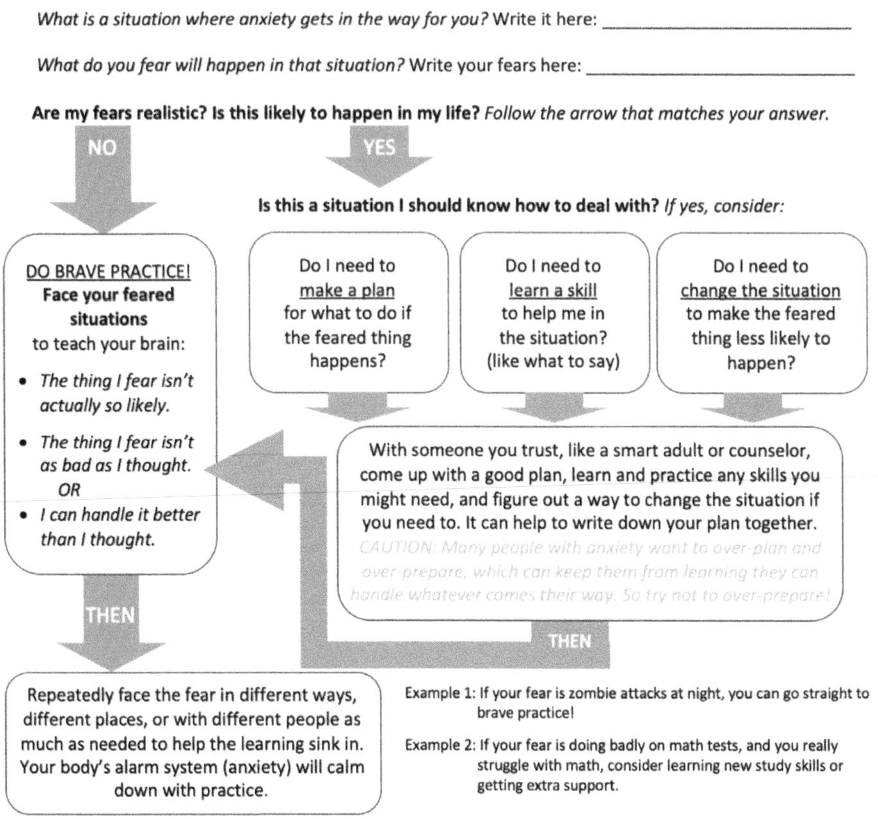

*What is a situation where anxiety gets in the way for you?* Write it here: _____

*What do you fear will happen in that situation?* Write your fears here: _____

**Are my fears realistic? Is this likely to happen in my life?** *Follow the arrow that matches your answer.*

NO          YES

**Is this a situation I should know how to deal with?** *If yes, consider:*

DO BRAVE PRACTICE!
**Face your feared situations**
to teach your brain:

- *The thing I fear isn't actually so likely.*
- *The thing I fear isn't as bad as I thought.* OR
- *I can handle it better than I thought.*

Do I need to make a plan for what to do if the feared thing happens?

Do I need to learn a skill to help me in the situation? (like what to say)

Do I need to change the situation to make the feared thing less likely to happen?

With someone you trust, like a smart adult or counselor, come up with a good plan, learn and practice any skills you might need, and figure out a way to change the situation if you need to. It can help to write down your plan together.

CAUTION: Many people with anxiety want to over-plan and over-prepare, which can keep them from learning they can handle whatever comes their way. So try not to over-prepare!

THEN

THEN

Repeatedly face the fear in different ways, different places, or with different people as much as needed to help the learning sink in. Your body's alarm system (anxiety) will calm down with practice.

Example 1: If your fear is zombie attacks at night, you can go straight to brave practice!

Example 2: If your fear is doing badly on math tests, and you really struggle with math, consider learning new study skills or getting extra support.

**Fig. 1.** Decision tree for using exposure to address fear of normal risk, age-appropriate situations.[37]

BHP should collaborate with the family to develop an exposure plan. Often, it is helpful for BHPs to set clear expectations for brief treatment, including session duration, meeting frequency, and total treatment length during the initial session with families. Starting this conversation early can help support efficient care transitions with families for whom additional community-based treatment is needed.

*Caregiver involvement in treatment:* Increasingly, evidence suggests that caregiver involvement is crucial for youth anxiety treatment, especially in the context of IPC. Specifically, caregivers can facilitate between-session exposures, and treatment may target specific caregiving behaviors that exacerbate anxiety, such as accommodation. Accommodation includes behaviors that caregivers use to decrease their

---

**Box 2**
**Resources for conducting exposures**

- Brief handouts for caregivers and youth: English, Spanish
- Workbooks to guide exposure-based treatment for children (English, Spanish) and adolescents (English and Spanish)
  ○ Includes key information and strategies that can be efficiently communicated to families

*Note:* Resources provided by First Approach Skills Training program.

child's anxiety or anxiety-related impairment, such as avoiding situations that may make their child anxious or removing their child from them or stepping in to perform a task for their child (eg, responding to questions directed at the child). Ideally, BHPs should aim to empower caregivers to understand the principles of exposure-based treatment so that they can independently support exposure practice and potentially reduce future recurrence. In some cases, caregivers' accommodation behaviors are an ideal treatment target, especially for young children. In the case of accommodation, BHPs can employ the principles of exposure practice to support caregivers in reducing accommodation behaviors.

*Case Presentation:* Below, the authors outline a fictionalized case example based on common presentations seen in IPC to illustrate a stepped approach to exposure-based anxiety intervention in primary care.

Tasha is an 8-year-old multiracial (White and Black) girl presenting in mid-September with recurrent stomach aches. The abdominal pain occurs each morning before school and sometimes during the day at school, frequently resulting in Tasha's father being called to pick Tasha up from school. No medical cause could be identified for Tasha's stomach discomfort. Tasha has a history of significant separation anxiety during her preschool years and was homeschooled for the last 2 years due to the COVID-19 pandemic. Tasha admits she feels nervous around peers, has difficulty making friends, and tends to play independently at recess. She denies any bullying or peer victimization. Otherwise, Tasha enjoys learning, does well academically, and wants to become a veterinarian when she's older.

After ruling out medical causes of Tasha's abdominal pain, Tasha's PCP referred Tasha and her family to brief behavioral intervention with the practice's BHP. During the initial appointment, the BHP met with Tasha's family to discuss their concerns and identify treatment priorities. Tasha shares that she often worries about what peers think of her and is nervous about starting conversations with new peers. Together, Tasha, her parents, and her clinician identify the following treatment goals: (1) increase the number of days Tasha can stay at school, (2) feel comfortable talking to new peers, and (3) make new friends. With those goals in mind, Tasha's family and her BHP discuss opportunities for exposure, which they call brave practice. Tasha's BHP also introduces additional parent strategies, including providing rewards for brave practice, validating Tasha when she feels anxious and expressing confidence in her ability to handle feared but typical situations (eg, recess) and encouraging Tasha to participate in regular activities even if anxiety is present (eg, recess).

Over the next few weeks, Tasha and her family implement structured brave practices. When possible, during the session, Tasha conducts brave practice with her BHP (eg, smiling at a peer in the waiting room), and otherwise the family uses session time to troubleshoot between-session practice and identify new opportunities for brave practice. Specific practices include (1) Tasha introducing herself and asking to play with children at a local park, (2) joining a new after-school club, and (3) participating in an open-invitation weekend meet-up with families of students in her class. Parents also identified accommodations they would begin to decrease, specifically speaking for Tasha in social situations (ordering food at restaurants, responding to questions from people she does not know well). At a 6-week follow-up appointment, Tasha and her parents reported less abdominal pain, no recent calls home, and Tasha said she had made friends.

*Pharmacotherapy for youth anxiety in primary care:* Pharmacotherapy treatment is outlined in accordance with the recommended sequence of care (**Boxes 3** and **4**) and is described in this elsewhere in this volume (see Pharmacotherapy for Pediatric Anxiety Disorders).

---

**Box 3**
**Psychoeducation about pharmacotherapy**

- It can take 6 weeks to see the full improvement of a given dose of medication, but improvement often starts in the first 2 weeks.

- It is important to plan how to consistently take these medications and discuss if you think it would be beneficial to have parental supervision of the doses to aid in consistency or safety. Fluoxetine may be a useful choice for teens without support from an adult to remember their medication due to the long half-life which prevents withdrawal symptoms from missed doses.

- Missed doses will lower the efficacy of the medication and at higher doses or with shorter acting agents can cause a withdrawal syndrome that include worsening anxiety and flu-like symptoms.

- Selective serotonin reuptake inhibitors and serotonin norepinephrine reuptake inhibitors are commonly well-tolerated (Mills and Strawn, 2020)[40]. Common adverse effects such as headaches, abdominal pain, restlessness, insomnia, and activation are typically most notable in the first 2 weeks of treatment and can trigger discontinuation if patients and parents are not aware these often improve.

- Children with anxiety, particularly at younger ages, are more likely to be sensitive to potential side effects, but starting at lower doses helps minimize the effects.

- Selective serotonin reuptake inhibitors and serotonin norepinephrine reuptake inhibitors can cause mood symptoms such as agitation, worsened anxiety, disinhibition, or suicidal ideation/self-harming behaviors. A discussion of the risk of suicidal thinking and behavior and the importance of close monitoring should be part of informed consent (see below).

- When teens or families are hesitant about these medications, providing a copy of the American Academy of Child and Adolescent Psychiatry (AACAPs) Anxiety Disorders Parents' Medication Guide (in English and Spanish) can be helpful to give to families to read prior to a follow-up appointment.[41]
    - https://www.aacap.org/App_Themes/AACAP/docs/resource_centers/resources/med_guides/anxiety-parents-medication-guide.pdf

---

## RECOMMENDATIONS
### *Selective-Serotonin Reuptake Inhibitors Dosing*

- Start at a low dose and titrate every 2 to 4 weeks until symptoms remit or side effects are emerging.[27]
- More recent data show that improvement emerges within 2 weeks of starting treatment and may occur more quickly with high-dose treatment compared with low dose.
- Selective-serotonin reuptake inhibitors (SSRIs) show a more rapid rate of improvement and overall greater magnitude of response compared with selective norepinephrine reuptake inhibitors (SNRIs).[28,29]
- If side effects are encountered, counsel patients regarding the transient nature of most side effects, but clinicians may choose to reduce the dose to minimize side effect risk.
- For prepubertal patients, decrease starting the dose by 1/2 and aim for 2/3 of the typical maximum dose for older patients.
- If symptoms are not controlled by the maximum tolerable dose, cross-taper to a second trail with an alternate SSRI.

### *Medication monitoring*

- Follow-up within 4 weeks after the initial dose is started, increase the dose every 4 weeks until significant improvement or side effects are encountered

---

**Box 4**
**Discussing boxed warning with families**

All serotonergic medications in the SSRI and SNRI families have a "boxed warning" from the US Food and Drug Administration. This warning was made in 2004 based on a meta-analysis of current research and states that there is increased risk of suicidal thinking and behavior for youth through age 24 years. In 2007, a meta-analysis was completed which included youth taking these medications for any indication. They reported that the risk of suicidal ideation for all youth with non-obsessive compulsive disorder (OCD) anxiety diagnoses was 1% for youth on an antidepressant compared with 0.2% for youth treated with placebo. The study found a small increased risk for suicidal ideation in the treatment groups (of 0.7%) with a number needed to harm of 143 compared with a number to a number needed to treat of 3. Clinically, suicidal thoughts seem most common when youth experience activation from an SSRI accompanied by increased emotional lability and impulsivity. Reassuringly, four subsequent meta-analyses of these medications in youth with anxiety disorders have failed to identify an increased incidence of suicidality.

*From* Suicidality in Children and Adolescents Being Treated with Antidepressant Medications and Bridge (2007).[38,39]

---

- More frequent contact if not in therapy, presence of depression or suicidal ideation, or concern for difficulty adhering to medication plan
- Track efficacy with repeated standardized measures such as the PROMIS Anxiety Short Form,[14] GAD-7 (youth 12 years and older),[30] Spence Children's Anxiety Scale,[31] or the Screen for Child Anxiety-Related Emotional Disorders[32]
- If no improvement, reconsider diagnosis, ask about frequency of missed doses, consider comorbid illness, inquire about substance use, and consider referral to psychiatric evaluation or consultation
- Most states now have a psychiatric consultant line: Check https://www.nnccap.org for a listing of consult lines in your state.[33]
- Once symptom remission is achieved, most patients benefit from continuing on the medication for 6 to 12 months to prevent relapse. During a period of stability, periodic attempts at discontinuation should be made with a gradual taper. If anxiety returns as the dose is lowered, slowing or reversing the taper can restabilize symptoms.[34]

### Discontinuing or changing medications

- For discontinuing: Consider decreasing the dose by 25% to 50% weekly to avoid withdrawal symptoms. Given the long half-life of fluoxetine, this may be of less concerns. For duloxetine and venlafaxine, both known for producing withdrawal effects, the taper rate may need to be more gradual.
- If switching to another medication, both conservative and more aggressive approaches have pros and cons:
  ○ Conservatively, tapering the first medication before starting a second medication reduces the risks of serotonin syndrome and other potential complications of taking two medications concurrently (eg, drug–drug interactions). This clarifies if side effects improve off of medication that they were drug related, but could lead to symptom exacerbation while under medication.
  ○ Conversely, cross-tapering over a period of 1 to 4 weeks onto a second medication, while still taking the first medication, exposes the patient to the potential adverse effects listed immediately above but decreases treatment interruption.

○ Directly switching off one medication onto a second medication is the least common strategy, but may be pursued if the first medication is causing significant adverse effects, the patient only recently started the first medication (eg, within last week), or the first medication has low potential for withdrawal if suddenly stopped (eg, low-dose fluoxetine)[35,36]

## Summary

Anxiety is a common mental health concern in pediatric primary care and rates are increasing. Fortunately, pediatric primary care settings are well situated to support early intervention for youth anxiety, including both behavioral and pharmacotherapy approaches. Effective behavioral intervention for anxiety should initiate exposure, or brave practice, as early as possible in treatment, with specific exposures derived from the youth's current functioning and the families' treatment priorities. Research in pharmacotherapy for pediatric anxiety supports SSRIs as a first-line treatment approach and SNRIs as a second-line approach due to higher side-effect burden. Pharmacotherapy interventions require careful consideration of dosing and comorbid conditions.

## CLINICS CARE POINTS

- Universal screening for youth anxiety in primary care using brief measures, such as the PROMIS Anxiety Short Form,[14] is recommended.
- Treatment for youth anxiety in primary care can include behavioral and pharmacotherapy approaches.
- Behavioral intervention for youth anxiety should prioritize early initiation of exposure practice.
- Caregivers' involvement in treatment is key for treatment effectiveness and reducing symptom recurrence.
- Selective-serotonin reuptake inhibitors are the first-line pharmacotherapy treatment approach for youth anxiety.
- Selective norepinephrine reuptake inhibitors may be a second-line pharmacotherapy treatment approach.

## AUTHOR DISCLOSURE STATEMENT

W.P. French receives clinical research support from the National Institute of Mental Health, United States. N. Jungbluth receives honoraria for providing trainings and consultation on integrated primary care topics. E. Dillon-Naftolin have nothing to disclose.

## REFERENCES

1. Merikangas KR, He JP, Burstein M, et al. Lifetime prevalence of mental disorders in us adolescents: results from the national comorbidity study-adolescent supplement (NCS-A). J Am Acad Child Adolesc Psychiatry 2010; 49(10):980-9.
2. Wehry AM, Beesdo-Baum K, Hennelly MM, et al. Assessment and treatment of anxiety disorders in children and adolescents. Curr Psychiatry Rep 2015; 17(7):1-11.

3. Bitsko RH, Holbrook JR, Ghandour RM, et al. Epidemiology and impact of health care provider–diagnosed anxiety and depression among US children. J Dev Behav Pediatr JDBP 2018;39(5):395.

4. Chavira DA, Ponting C, Ramos G. The impact of COVID-19 on child and adolescent mental health and treatment considerations. Behav Res Ther 2022;104169. https://doi.org/10.1016/j.brat.2022.104169.

5. Brown JD, Wissow LS, Zachary C, et al. Receiving advice about child mental health from a primary care provider: african American and Hispanic parent attitudes. Med Care 2007;45:1076–82.

6. Arora PG, Godoy L, Hodgkinson S. Serving the underserved: cultural considerations in behavioral health integration in pediatric primary care. Prof Psychol Res Pr 2017;48(3):139.

7. Hodgkinson S, Godoy L, Beers LS, et al. Improving mental health access for low-income children and families in the primary care setting. Pediatrics 2017; 139(1):1–9.

8. Cohen E, Calderon E, Salinas G, et al. Parents' perspectives on access to child and adolescent mental health services. Soc Work Ment Health 2012;10(4): 294–310.

9. Barlow M, Wildman B, Stancin T. Mothers' help-seeking for pediatric psychosocial problems. Clin Pediatr (Phila) 2005;44(2):161–7.

10. Chavira DA, Stein MB, Bailey K, et al. Child anxiety in primary care: prevalent but untreated. Depress Anxiety 2004;20(4):155–64.

11. Asarnow JR, Rozenman M, Wiblin J, et al. Integrated medical-behavioral care compared with usual primary care for child and adolescent behavioral health: a meta-analysis. JAMA Pediatr 2015;169(10):929–37.

12. Kolko DJ, Campo J, Kilbourne AM, et al. Collaborative care outcomes for pediatric behavioral health problems: a cluster randomized trial. Pediatrics 2014;133(4): e981–92.

13. Mangione CM, Barry MJ, Nicholson WK, et al. US Preventive Services Task Force, Screening for anxiety in children and adolescents: US preventive services task force recommendation statement. JAMA 2022;328(14):1438.

14. Varni JW, Magnus B, Stucky BD, et al. Psychometric properties of the PROMIS® pediatric scales: precision, stability, and comparison of different scoring and administration options. Qual Life Res 2014;23(4):1233–43.

15. Hacker KA, Penfold R, Arsenault L, et al. Screening for behavioral health issues in children enrolled in Massachusetts Medicaid. Pediatrics 2014;133(1):46–54.

16. Rushton J, Bruckman D, Kelleher K. Primary care referral of children with psychosocial problems. Arch Pediatr Adolesc Med 2002;156(6):592–8.

17. Silk JS, Tan PZ, Ladouceur CD, et al. A randomized clinical trial comparing individual cognitive behavioral therapy and child-centered therapy for child anxiety disorders. J Clin Child Adolesc Psychol 2016;1–13. https://doi.org/10.1080/15374416.2016.1138408.

18. Whiteside SP, Sim LA, Morrow AS, et al. A meta-analysis to guide the enhancement of CBT for childhood anxiety: exposure over anxiety management. Clin Child Fam Psychol Rev 2020;23(1):102–21.

19. James A, James G, Cowdrey F, et al. Cognitive behaviour therapy for anxiety disorders in children and adolescents. Cochrane Database Syst Rev 2015;11: CD004690.

20. Keeton CP, Caporino NE, Kendall PC, et al. Mood and suicidality outcomes 3–11 years following pediatric anxiety disorder treatment. Depress Anxiety 2019; 36(10):930–40.

21. Zhang H, Zhang Y, Yang L, et al. Efficacy and acceptability of psychotherapy for anxious young children: a meta-analysis of randomized controlled trials. J Nerv Ment Dis 2017;205(12):931–41.

22. Merikangas KR, He JP, Burstein M, et al. Service utilization for lifetime mental disorders in US adolescents: results of the National Comorbidity Survey–Adolescent Supplement (NCS-A). J Am Acad Child Adolesc Psychiatry 2011;50(1):32–45.

23. Kozlowski JL, Lusk P, Melnyk BM. Pediatric nurse practitioner management of child anxiety in a rural primary care clinic with the evidence-based COPE program. J Pediatr Health Care 2015;29(3):274–82.

24. Ginsburg GS, Drake KL, Winegrad H, et al. An open trial of the Anxiety Action Plan (AxAP): a brief pediatrician-delivered intervention for anxious youth. Child Youth Care Forum 2016;45:19–32. Springer.

25. Peris TS, Compton SN, Kendall PC, et al. Trajectories of change in youth anxiety during cognitive behavior therapy. J Consult Clin Psychol 2015;83(2):239–52.

26. Craske MG, Treanor M, Zbozinek TD, et al. Optimizing exposure therapy with an inhibitory retrieval approach and the OptEx Nexus. Behav Res Ther 2022;152:104069.

27. Kodish I, Rockhill C, Varley C. Pharmacotherapy for anxiety disorders in children and adolescents. Dialogues Clin Neurosci 2022;13:439–52.

28. Strawn JR, Mills JA, Cornwall GJ, et al. Buspirone in children and adolescents with anxiety: a review and Bayesian analysis of abandoned randomized controlled trials. J Child Adolesc Psychopharmacol 2018;28(1):2–9.

29. Strawn JR, Prakash A, Zhang Q, et al. A randomized, placebo-controlled study of duloxetine for the treatment of children and adolescents with generalized anxiety disorder. J Am Acad Child Adolesc Psychiatry 2015;54(4):283–93.

30. Mossman SA, Luft MJ, Schroeder HK, et al. The generalized anxiety disorder 7-item (GAD-7) scale in adolescents with generalized anxiety disorder: signal detection and validation. Ann Clin Psychiatry 2017;29(4):227–234A.

31. Spence SH. Spence children's anxiety scale. J Anxiety Disord 1997.

32. Birmaher B, Khetarpal S, Brent D, et al. The screen for child anxiety related emotional disorders (SCARED): scale construction and psychometric characteristics. J Am Acad Child Adolesc Psychiatry 1997;36(4):545–53.

33. NNCPAP national network of child psychiatry access programs. NNCPAP national network of child psychiatry access programs. Available at: https://www.nncpap.org. Accessed December 13, 2022.

34. Pine DS. Treating children and adolescents with selective serotonin reuptake inhibitors: how long is appropriate? J Child Adolesc Psychopharmacol 2002;12(3):189–203.

35. Walter HJ, Bukstein OG, Abright AR, et al. Clinical practice guideline for the assessment and treatment of children and adolescents with anxiety disorders. J Am Acad Child Adolesc Psychiatry 2020;59(10):1107–24.

36. Ogle NR, Akkerman SR. Guidance for the discontinuation or switching of antidepressant therapies in adults. J Pharm Pract 2013;26(4):389–96.

37. Jungbluth N, Read KL, Blossom JB. First Approach Skills Training for Youth Anxiety (FAST-A): Workbook. Published online 2021.

38. Research C for DE. Suicidality in children and adolescents being treated with antidepressant medications. FDA. 2018. Available at: https://www.fda.gov/drugs/postmarket-drug-safety-information-patients-and-providers/suicidality-children-and-adolescents-being-treated-antidepressant-medications. Accessed December 13, 2022.

39. Bridge JA, Iyengar S, Salary CB, et al. Clinical response and risk for reported suicidal ideation and suicide attempts in pediatric antidepressant treatment: a meta-analysis of randomized controlled trials. JAMA 2007;297(15):1683–96.
40. Mills JA, Strawn JR. Antidepressant tolerability in pediatric anxiety and obsessive-compulsive disorders: a Bayesian hierarchical modeling meta-analysis. J Am Acad Child Adolesc Psychiatry 2020;59(11):1240–51.
41. American Academy of. Child and Adolescent Psychiatry. Anxiety disorders: Parents' Medication Guide 2020;1–20.

# Social Media and Anxiety in Youth

## A Narrative Review and Clinical Update

Megan D. Chochol, MD[a],*, Kriti Gandhi, MD[b],
Paul E. Croarkin, DO, MS[c]

### KEYWORDS

- Adolescents • Anxiety • Children • Social media • Facebook • FOMO
- Generalized anxiety disorder • Instagram

### KEY POINTS

- Social media use and related research focused on the child and adolescent mental health continues to evolve rapidly.
- Social media's impact and relationship with anxiety has been understudied.
- We examined relevant systematic and narrative reviews.
- Duration, frequency, and type of social media use may have correlations with anxiety.
- Further research focused on anxiety and social media is urgently needed.

There are ongoing concerns about the effects of social media on adolescent mental health. Few earlier studies have examined social media in the context of anxiety. This review provides background on social media use in youth through developmental and neurobiological lenses, summarizes recent systematic reviews and meta-analyses, then narrative reviews on anxiety and social media use offer guidance on how to best address social media use in youth, and suggests future directions for research and clinical practice.

## WHAT IS SOCIAL MEDIA, AND HOW HAS IT EVOLVED OVER THE YEARS?

The definition of "social media" varies, and social media continues to evolve rapidly. Social media includes Internet-based platforms that rely on user-generated content comprising user-specific profiles maintained by the platform. Ultimately, social media

[a] Department of Psychiatry, University of Utah and Huntsman Mental Health Institute, 501 Chipeta Way, Salt Lake City, UT 84108, USA; [b] Department of Psychiatry, Children's National Hospital, Takoma Theatre, 6833 4th Street NW, Washington, DC 20012, USA; [c] Department of Psychiatry and Psychology, Mayo Clinic, 200 First Street SW, Rochester, MN 55902, USA
* Corresponding author.
*E-mail address:* megan.chochol@hsc.utah.edu

Child Adolesc Psychiatric Clin N Am 32 (2023) 613–630
https://doi.org/10.1016/j.chc.2023.02.004
1056-4993/23/© 2023 Elsevier Inc. All rights reserved.
**childpsych.theclinics.com**

platforms connect users, facilitating the development of social networks.[1] Over time, they have adapted to usage trends, shifting toward more concise and visual content and expanding their reach to broader audiences.

The evolving definition of social media and the need for a well-operationalized definition of social media use complicates research on the topic. Social media use commonly focuses on the amount of time one spends engaging with social media; however, researchers have conceptualized it in various ways. Most fundamentally, social media engagement has been separated dichotomously into active use, generating and reacting to content, versus passive use, consuming content as an observer. More nuanced types of social media engagement have also been described.[2–4]

### IT FEELS LIKE TIMES ARE CHANGING, BUT WHAT ARE THE DATA ON SOCIAL MEDIA USE IN YOUTH?

YouTube is currently the most used social media platform by adolescents aged 13 to 17 years (95% endorsed ever using Youtube), followed by TikTok (67%), and Instagram (32%).[5] Internet usage trends show an increase from 24% of teens endorsing almost constant Internet use in 2014 to 2015 to 46% of teens in 2022.[5] There are demographic and socioeconomic status differences in social media use. Black and Hispanic teens (56% and 55%, respectively) are significantly more likely than White teens (37%) to constantly use the Internet, and teens in low-income households are more likely to use Facebook.[5] The onset of the COVID-19 pandemic in December 2019 was associated with an increased media use for various purposes.[6] As usage trends have increased, anxiety, depression, suicide attempts, and suicide completions over time in children and adolescents have increased[7–10] fueling concerns about a link (**Fig. 1, Fig. 2**).

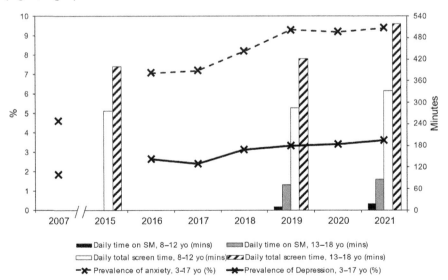

**Fig. 1.** Annual depression, anxiety, and social media use trends. Daily time on SM, 8–12 yo: 2019 – 10 min, 2021 – 18 min. Daily time on SM, 13–18 yo: 2019 – 70 min, 2021 – 87 min. Daily total screen time, 8–12 yo: 2015 – 276 min, 2019 – 284 min, 2021 – 333 min. Daily total screen time, 13–18 yo: 2015 – 400 min, 2019 – 422 min, 2021 – 519 min. Anxiety and depression data source: https://www.census.gov/programs-surveys/nsch/data/datasets.html. Social media use data source: https://www.commonsensemedia.org/sites/default/files/research/report/8-18-census-integrated-report-final-web_0.pdf.

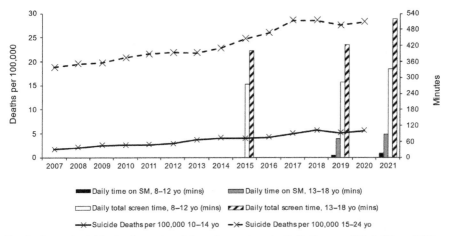

**Fig. 2.** Annual suicide deaths and social media use trends. Daily time on SM, 8–12 yo: 2019 – 10 min, 2021 – 18 min. Daily time on SM, 13–18 yo: 2019–70 min, 2021–87 min. Daily total screen time, 8–12 yo: 2015 – 276 min, 2019 – 284 min, 2021 – 333 min. Daily total screen time, 13–18 yo: 2015 – 400 min, 2019 – 422 min, 2021 – 519 min. Suicide deaths data source: https://www.cdc.gov/nchs/data/databriefs/db433-tables.pdf#2. Social media use data source: https://www.commonsensemedia.org/sites/default/files/research/report/8-18-census-integrated-report-final-web_0.pdf.

Accordingly, new assessment tools and mental health disorders are being proposed. Problematic social media use refers to a pattern of social media engagement despite problematic consequences resulting in addiction-like symptoms.[11] Internet Gaming Disorder is described and recommended for further research in the Diagnostic and Statistical Manual of Mental Disorders, Fifth Edition (DSM-5). Although it has not yet been recognized as an independent disorder in the DSM-5, the criteria have been extrapolated to describe other Specific Internet Use Disorders as defined by the International Classification of Diseases-11 separate from gaming disorders.[12]

## HOW DO WE LOOK AT SOCIAL MEDIA USE IN YOUTH THROUGH A DEVELOPMENTAL LENS?

Child and adolescent developmental processes can unfold or derail on social media platforms. Age-based windows where correlations exist between social media use and well-being/ill-being suggest developmental underpinnings.[13] For example, very-high and very-low social media use correlate with lower life satisfaction ratings in older adolescents (aged 16–21 years). In younger adolescents (aged 10–15 years), a more linear relationship was found with increasing use, along with lower life satisfaction ratings in girls compared with boys.[13] There were differences in the age-based sensitivity windows for male adolescents (aged 14–15 years and 19 years) and female adolescents (aged 11–13 years and 19 years). Furthermore, a sex-based bidirectional inverse relationship between social media use and well-being during specific ages of adolescence was also found.[13]

Adolescents cultivate trust in social relationships through self-disclosure. There was a positive bidirectional relationship between adolescent self-disclosure and psychological well-being[14] and potential benefit from social media use in adolescence on developing empathy and improvements in self-esteem and well-being.[15] Additionally, the strength of the relationship between 2 individuals correlates with how happy one feels after reading a positive Facebook post about the other.[16] Although adolescents preferred face-to-face communication, online self-disclosure positively influenced initiation of offline friendships and can be helpful for those with social anxiety.[14]

Adolescents are arguably more susceptible to social pressures, including the tendency to imitate an observed behavior. Research is growing on this contagion effect within social media use, for example, with respect to suicide and tics.[17,18] Youth are more likely to "like" popular content with many "likes" than less popular content.[19] Furthermore, experimental modification of an individual's Facebook news feed alters the individual's posting behaviors accordingly.[16]

## HOW DO WE LOOK AT SOCIAL MEDIA USE IN YOUTH THROUGH A NEUROBIOLOGICAL LENS?

White matter connections increase during adolescence, improving communication between brain structures and increasing behavioral and emotional regulation. Simultaneously, gray matter volume decreases, notably in areas involved in social engagement.[20] The incomplete development of the prefrontal and parietal cortices involved in executive functioning and emotional regulatory networks may result in adolescents being more vulnerable to emotional social media content and the potential negative consequences of social media use,[20,21] just because they are more susceptible to social pressures offline.

Greater activation of reward circuitry correlates with receiving "likes" on personal content and when viewing others' content with many likes.[19] Viewing popular content was also associated with activation in brain areas involved in visual attention.[19] Activation of brain areas involved in providing social support is related to "liking" content. These neurobiological circuits evolved in primates and humans as social engagement deepened, and their implication in social media use may foster positive social development.[22] Regarding cognition, a recent study on more than 12,000 adolescents, including a portion with problematic social media use, showed no significant correlation between social media use on various domains of cognition.[23]

## SUMMARY OF RESULTS OF SYSTEMATIC REVIEWS AND META-ANALYSES

A broad search of PubMed using the terms "anxiety" and "social media" identified 6 relevant systematic reviews and meta-analyses. A seventh systematic review was included based on review of the references (**Table 1**). The fact that our search for studies resulted in 7 systematic reviews and meta-analyses from the past 5 years with little overlap in included studies underscores the heterogeneity of research and recent productive study of the role of social media in adolescent mental health.

Shannon and colleagues systematically examined associations between problematic social media use and mental health outcomes, including depressive symptoms, anxiety symptoms, and stress. Eighteen studies from the United States, Europe, the Middle East, and Asia included study populations aged 12 to 30 years and used validated scales. The association between problematic social media use and anxiety was weak (r = 0.348, $P < .001$), and heterogeneity was greatest in anxiety assessments. There were also weak correlations between problematic social media use and depression (r = 0.273, $P < .001$) and stress (r = 0.313, $P < .001$) with no heterogeneity based on age, gender, or year of publication.[24]

Alonzo and colleagues systematically reviewed the relationship between active Internet use, sleep quality, and mental health outcomes, including anxiety, depression, and psychological distress, using validated scales in individuals aged 12 to 30 years across many countries. They assessed these variables as potential mediators,

**Table 1**
Systematic Reviews and Meta-Analyses on Social Media and Anxiety in Youth from the Past 5 Years (2018–2022)

| Author, Year | Title | Study Type | N | Age |
|---|---|---|---|---|
| Hancock et al,[4] 2022 | Psychological well-being and social media use: a meta-analysis of associations between social media use and depression, anxiety, loneliness, eudaimonic, hedonic, and social well-being | MA and NR | 226 studies | Adolescent and older |
| Shannon et al,[24] 2022 | Problematic Social Media Use in Adolescents and Young Adults: Systematic Review and Meta-analysis | SR and MA | 18 studies; 9269 subjects | 12–30 yo |
| Alonzo et al,[26] 2021 | Interplay between social media use, sleep quality, and mental health in youth: A systematic review | SR | 42 studies | 12–30 yo |
| Piteo et al,[27] 2020 | Review: Social networking sites and associations with depressive and anxiety symptoms in children and adolescents – a systematic review | SR and MA | 19 studies | 5–18 yo |
| Cataldo et al, 2020 | Social Media Usage and Development of Psychiatric Disorders in Childhood and Adolescence: A Review | SR | 44 studies | 10–19 yo |
| Marino et al,[29] 2018 | The associations between problematic Facebook use, psychological distress and well-being among adolescents and young adults: A systematic review and meta-analysis | SR and MA | 23 studies; 13,929 subjects | 16.5–32.4 yo |
| Hussain and Griffiths[30] 2018 | Problematic Social Networking Site Use and Comorbid Psychiatric Disorders: A Systematic Review of Recent Large-Scale Studies | SR | 9 studies | 12–88 yo |

*Abbreviations:* MA, meta-analysis; SR, systematic review; yo, years old.
A table of key elements of systematic reviews and meta-analyses on social media and anxiety in youth from the past 5 years organized in chronological order.

moderators, or confounders of the relationship. Of the 42 studies included, only 7 focused on social media use, whereas the rest evaluated general Internet use. Of these 7 studies, only 3 described findings on anxiety—increased time spent on social media correlated with higher anxiety levels. One study found this association only when perceived consequences were not considered, suggesting that acknowledgment of consequences plays a role in outcome.[25] When looking at the presence or absence of smartphone-interrupted sleep, there was no correlation with mental health symptoms, and most smartphone-interrupted sleep was due to text messages rather than social media use. There was evidence that poor sleep quality mediates the relationship between Internet/smartphone/social media use and poor mental health outcomes in youth.[26]

Piteo and Ward examined relationships between social media use and depression and anxiety symptoms in 19 studies with participants aged 5 to 18 years across Asia, North America, Australia, and Europe. Included studies assessed not only time spent on social media but also the type of use and specific platforms, and outcomes were assessed using validated instruments. Again, correlations between time on social media use and increased anxiety symptoms were weak. The number of social media accounts correlated moderately with increased anxiety symptoms, although the sample size was small, and the frequency of checking social media accounts correlated weakly with increased anxiety. Fear of missing out (FOMO) was a mediating variable and perceived social support and social comparison were postulated to affect the relationship between social media use and symptoms of depression and anxiety.[27]

Cataldo and colleagues provided an overview of correlations between problematic social media use with cognitive, psychological, and social outcomes in 44 studies, including youth aged 10 to 19 years. Correlations between social media use and anxiety ranged from insignificant to moderate. There was a direct association between addictive social media use behaviors, increased anxiety, and poorer academic performance.[28] Social anxiety correlated with behavioral dimensions, for example, comparing one's own photo with others' pictures on social media platforms. A direct link was found between Instagram use and anxiety in boys, whereas in girls, body image dissatisfaction mediated this link suggesting different mechanisms at play in each gender. One prospective study found that using Facebook at 17 years of age to alleviate boredom predicted increased anxiety at age 19, suggesting anxiety may be a product of social media use. The authors speculated that increased unstructured time and decreased adult oversight after graduating high school may play a role and that those with a predisposition to anxiety may be more prone to problematic social media use, which may cyclically reinforce and perpetuate anxiety.[28]

Marino and colleagues focused on problematic Facebook use. They included 23 studies with participants aged 16.5 to 32.4 years. There were weak correlations between problematic Facebook use and psychological distress, with correlation coefficients ranging from 0.23 to 0.34 and a corrected mean correlation coefficient for anxiety of 0.33. Higher mean age and population samples from Western countries were associated more strongly with measures of psychological distress. There were also weak negative correlations between problematic Facebook use and well-being, with a corrected mean correlation coefficient of −0.22.[29]

Hussain and Griffiths reviewed 9 large-scale studies (N > 500) on social media use and comorbid psychiatric disorders. Study populations ranged from 12 to 88 years old, although most were limited to adolescents and young adults. Six studies specifically assessed anxiety, effect sizes were weak, and there was notable heterogeneity in anxiety metrics across studies. Five studies excluded for inadequate sample sizes also found a positive correlation between problematic social media use and anxiety.[30]

Hancock and colleagues explored associations between social media use and multiple mental health outcomes, including depression, anxiety, loneliness, and 3 dimensions of well-being: eudaimonic, hedonic, and social well-being. They included 226 quantitative studies with populations of adolescents and older published between 2006 and 2018. They defined theoretical, methodological, and study-level moderators for data analysis. There was no significant relationship between social media use and well-being as a single dimension, but effect sizes did vary across moderators. There was a weak correlation between social media use and anxiety ($r = 0.13$, $P < .01$) but no association between the 2 in longitudinal studies (only positive associations between social media use and depression and social well-being). Additionally, there was no difference in anxiety between active and passive social media use, even though active but not passive use was associated with general well-being, eudaimonic well-being, and social well-being. Further analyses found no directional, causal relationships between outcomes. The positive effect on well-being seems to be related to the social support derived from social media use, especially related to self-disclosure.[4]

## SUMMARY OF RESULTS OF NARRATIVE REVIEWS

Our search returned ten narrative reviews; an eleventh was included based on a review of references (**Table 2**). These reviews included studies from many countries and a wide range of participant ages, although most subjects were adolescents and college-age youth. There was significant heterogeneity across reviews with respect to the types of Internet, phone, and social media use included, as well as the mental health outcomes explored. Here, we focus on the results related to anxiety and social media use.

**Table 2**
**Narrative Reviews on Social Media and Anxiety in Youth from the Past 5 Years (2018–2022)**

| Author, Year | Title |
| --- | --- |
| Primack et al,[16] 2022 | Social Media as It Interfaces with Psychosocial Development and Mental Illness in Transitional-Age Youth |
| Kovačić Petrović et al,[36] 2022 | Internet use and internet-based addictive behaviors during coronavirus pandemic |
| Glover et al,[6] 2022 | #KidsAnxiety and the Digital World |
| Beyens et al,[33] 2022 | Social Media, parenting, and well-being |
| Haddad et al,[37] 2021 | The Impact of Social Media on College Mental Health During the COVID-19 Pandemic: a Multinational Review of the Existing Literature |
| Sarmiento et al,[35] 2020 | How Does Social Media Use Relate to Adolescents' Internalizing Symptoms? Conclusions from a Systematic Narrative Review |
| Zdanowicz et al,[38] 2020 | Screen Time and Belgian Teenagers |
| Steele et al,[21] 2020 | Conceptualizing digital stress in adolescents and young adults: toward the development of an empirically based model |
| Odgers and Jensen[34] 2020 | Annual Research Review: Adolescent Mental Health in the Digital Age: Facts, Fears and Future Directions |
| Mougharbel and Goldfield[31] 2020 | Psychological Correlates of Sedentary Screen Time Behavior Among Children and Adolescents: A Narrative Review |
| Ghaemi et al,[32] 2020 | Digital depression: a new disease of the millennium? |

A table of key elements of narrative reviews on social media and anxiety in youth from the past 5 years organized in chronological order.

Three larger population studies revealed positive correlations between increased social media use and anxiety, problematic Facebook use and social anxiety, and symptoms of anxiety, OCD, and potentially addictive use of social media.[16] Social media use and screen time were associated with poorer mental health outcomes in children and adolescents.[31,32] There is a potential association between social media use and increased multitasking, independently linked to decreased attention, academic performance, subjective well-being, and increased depression and anxiety.[16] Socially anxious youth seeking external validation are at greater risk for problematic Internet use.[6] Notably, active parental mediation and an autonomy-supportive parenting style around social media use correlated with fewer anxiety and depressive symptoms in youth and fewer depressive symptoms in youth experiencing cyberbullying.[33]

Overall, associations between the quantity of digital technology use and mental health outcomes, including anxiety, are inconsistent and small. There was no support for causality on analysis and little evidence to support an association between adolescent mental health outcomes and social media use at the population level.[34] Longitudinal studies provide some evidence that anxiety induces changes in adolescent social media use patterns, yet there is no evidence for the reverse.[35] The way variables, outcomes, and confounders were defined produced a wide variety of effect sizes and unreliable conclusions, highlighting the need for further studies exploring moderating and mediating factors.[34,35]

During the COVID-19 pandemic, the prevalence of anxiety was found to be 26.4% in one population, with a corresponding social media addiction prevalence of 6.8%. Overall, Internet addiction and problematic smartphone use were higher in youth during the pandemic. However, a Chinese study found that use was higher early in the pandemic compared with one and a half months later.[36,37] Anxiety correlated with frequent Internet and technology use among adolescents and adults,[6] problematic Internet use was a risk factor for Internet addiction.[36] The correlations between social media use and anxiety during the pandemic found in Chinese population samples were not found in a population sample from the Netherlands,[37] suggesting unrecognized moderating factors at play. Additionally, a fear of COVID-19 in Italian students during the first pandemic lockdown was linked to Internet addiction and higher rates of anxiety.[36] At the same time, COVID stress moderated the relationship between social media use and depression symptoms but not anxiety symptoms in a Chinese population.[37]

Few studies have explored specific social media platforms. Most have focused on Facebook, and a correlation was found between youth with insecure attachment and higher Facebook use.[38] One population-based survey ranked changes in depression and anxiety symptoms after social media use by platform from most to least detrimental: Instagram, Snapchat, Facebook, and Twitter.[32]

Female gender was more strongly associated with increased social media use greater than 3.5 hours per week and social media addiction compared with male gender.[36] There is some evidence that girls are more susceptible to the impact of social anxiety on social media use.[35] Additionally, female adolescents and youth with lower online popularity were more sensitive to the effects of approval anxiety, including depressive symptoms.[21] Nevertheless, male gender was associated with social media addiction during the COVID-19 pandemic.[36]

FOMO correlates with lower mood and lower life satisfaction.[21] Additionally, FOMO moderates and mediates social media use itself, ambivalence toward social media use, online communication patterns, and negative consequences of social media use, including symptoms of anxiety, depression, and a need to "belong" and for "popularity," among others.[21] In fact, FOMO-driven social media use is a risk factor for suicide.[38] Concerning anxiety, FOMO has been found to mediate the relationship between anxiety and negative consequences in youth. There is an association between youth with high anxiety and high cooccurring levels of FOMO and problematic social media use.[6] Youth may use social media as an unhealthy coping mechanism, inadvertently fostering corumination and avoidance, which can further exacerbate anxiety in a positive-feedback loop.[6,38]

## DOES SOCIAL MEDIA USE CAUSE POORER MENTAL HEALTH OUTCOMES IN YOUTH?

Overall, the evidence supporting the hypothesis that social media use may detrimentally affect youth mental health is correlational and weak. There is also correlational and weak evidence to support the hypothesis that social media use may beneficially affect youth mental health. It is essential to recognize that the evidence is mixed when discussing social media use with patients and families to avoid perpetuating a potentially inaccurate confirmation bias. For example, the Monitoring the Future Study in the United States strongly concluded that digital technology use was linked to depression[39]; however, reanalyses of the data showed results were highly dependent on modeling and confounding variables.[34]

Accordingly, methodology must be carefully considered. Studies relied almost exclusively on cross-sectional design, correlational data, and self-reported data subject to recall bias. Compounding this, framing social media use as addictive in a study provokes more negative responses related to well-being.[4] Variables and terms related to social media use are poorly defined, and screen time as a measure of social media use rather than type or style limits the ability to assess outcomes. Without well-operationalized terms and variables, there is a lack of assessment tools for research, resulting in heterogeneity in research methods. Methodology must also be flexible enough to adapt as social media platforms evolve.

The lack of adequate consideration of confounding, mediating, and moderating variables was one of the most notable limitations of the literature, and most studies acknowledged this. We conceptualize potential moderating and mediating variables in 5 categories: biological, psychological, social, investigational, and social media use (**Fig. 3**) and provide a nonexhaustive list of variables for consideration (**Table 3**). A high-quality research methodology that addresses the current limitations, especially potential moderating and mediating factors, is needed to understand better the links between social media use and mental health in youth.

Generalizability is also a limitation. Population samples were biased toward adolescents rather than children, and community samples rather than clinical populations. Generalizability between social media platforms or even within the same platform at a later time may be limited, given how quickly they evolve. Additionally, results may be specific to the cultures and geographic regions in which they were studied. For example, associations differed between adolescents, adults, and college students[4] and between Western and Asian populations.[4,37] Furthermore, results obtained during the COVID-19 pandemic may not be generalizable to future time frames.

In addition to the potentially harmful effects of social media use on mental health, there are other risks to consider. Social media use may expose youth to inappropriate content and cyberbullying, which is more detrimental than offline bullying with respect to mental health, including suicidal ideation, physical health, self-esteem, and absenteeism.[40] Additionally, social media engagement is ripe for misinformation and personal data exploitation.[41] Youth are creating a permanent digital footprint during a developmental period when they inherently cannot appreciate the potential long-term consequences of posting content on future academic and career opportunities.

Although most study hypotheses speculate social media use contributes adversely to mental health in youth, one can imagine favorable impacts, too. Social media

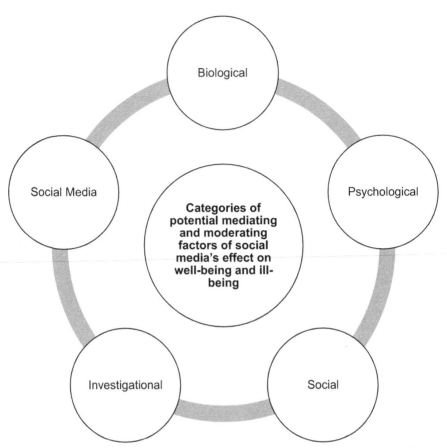

**Fig. 3.** Categories of potential mediating and moderating factors of social media's effect on well-being and ill-being.

provides a setting where adolescents can explore their identity, experiment with self-disclosure, and practice social skills. Through online engagement, they can enhance offline relationships and form meaningful online relationships. More broadly, social media has the potential to reduce mental health stigma, provide social support, expand access to educational and mental health information, and even promote treatment.[6] Social media platforms may provide a more accessible source of support networks for those struggling with anxiety.[6] YouTube use was associated with beneficial mental health outcomes[32] and increased texting in adolescents at risk for substance use and externalizing problems correlated with less same-day anxiety.[34] More research is needed on the potential for positive impacts of social media.

## HOW SHOULD CAREGIVERS AND CLINICIANS PROCEED?

National organizations, including the American Academy of Child and Adolescent Psychiatry and the American Academy of Pediatrics, published online guidance for parents and caregivers on managing social media use. Specifically, concerning anxiety, they advise limiting the use of social media, which enables avoidance and perpetuates anxiety. Furthermore, families can use social media as a reward for youth avoiding

**Table 3**
**Categories of Potential Mediating and Moderating Factors of Social Media's Effect on Well-Being and Ill-Being with a Nonexhaustive List of Examples**

| Biological | Psychological | Social | Investigational | Social Media |
|---|---|---|---|---|
| Chronological age | Personality traits | Socio-demographic background | Methodology from study design to data analysis | Type of engagement |
| Developmental age | Resilience and coping skills | Cultural background | Framing | Type of communication |
| Developmental stages (physical, cognitive, social and emotional, moral) | Susceptibility to digital stress | Family dynamics | Operationalization of SM-related terms and outcomes | Frequency of use |
| Sex and gender | FOMO | Parenting styles | Biases | Total time of use |
| Genetics | Attachment style | Social support | | Platform(s) used |
| Family history of medical of mental health disorders | Self-esteem | Social engagement | | Parental oversight |
| Personal history of medical or mental health disorders | Values | Discrimination | | |
| Activity level | Hx of psychological trauma | Bullying | | |
| Nutrition | | Hobbies and activities | | |
| Sleep | | Widespread public issues (pandemics, climate change, politics, war) | | |
| | | Local public issues | | |

*Abbreviations:* FOMO, fear of missing out; Hx, history; SM–social media.

Conceptualization of categories of potential mediating and moderating factors of social media's effect on well-being and ill-being with a nonexhaustive list of examples important to consider in future research.

school or offline social engagement[6] and can limit time on social media if clinical concerns are present.[32]

Parental mediating and moderating of social media use have the potential to decrease ill-being along a variety of metrics, including anxiety.[33] These techniques can be implemented in styles that echo parenting literature.[33] We suspect, similar to conclusions in the parenting literature that a more authoritative style is most effective in maximizing positive benefits and minimizing the negative impacts of social media use.

Many concerned caregivers turn to clinicians for guidance. Social media use in youth is so prevalent that it has been suggested that the widely used HEADSSS (Home, Education & Employment, Activities, Drugs, Sex, Suicide, Safety) assessment be updated to HEADS4 (Home, Education & Employment, Activities, Drugs, Sex, Suicide, Safety, Social media use) to include social media use.[42] Assessment of problematic social media use should be based on a comprehensive clinical interview and the use of validated assessment tools. The PQRST (Provocation, Quality, Radiation/Region, Severity, Timing) pain assessment tool can be adapted to guide the clinical interview (**Table 4**). The most commonly used assessment tools for problematic use of social media are based on addiction literature, outdated, do not consider different and evolving social media platforms, and need updating.[43]

In patients with suspected or identified problematic social media use, and comorbid physical and mental health disorders, including poor sleep,[44] should be identified and their management optimized.[42] Pharmacotherapy data for Internet use disorders are limited. There is some evidence to support escitalopram, citalopram, bupropion, olanzapine, quetiapine, naltrexone, and memantine,[42] although this may be tied to the treatment of underlying comorbid mental health disorders.

The data on therapy treatment modalities are also mixed, and studies vary in quality. Still, cognitive behavioral therapy (CBT) and acceptance and commitment therapy (ACT) approaches, offline social skills development, group counseling, and sports interventions have some evidence as potential therapeutic modalities for problematic social media use. Steele's 4 components of digital stress (availability stress, approval anxiety, FOMO, and connection overload) could help guide therapy treatment planning.[21] Additionally, therapy can bolster skills that may beneficially affect associations between social media use and poor mental health effects, including optimistic thinking, mindfulness, cognitive reappraisal abilities, and dialectical thinking.[37] Higher levels of care specializing in Internet use disorders include multidisciplinary clinics, inpatient programs, residential programs, and wilderness programs.[42] Evidence for abstinence from social media use is mixed[21] and may not be possible given its prevalence. That said, establishing social media-free times may be helpful.[44]

Technology-based treatment modalities are increasing but there is little research on their efficacy. Increasing evidence supports structured CBT-based interventions that are delivered online.[6] Interventions delivered to youth via social media sites showed no benefit in anxiety symptoms despite improvement in depressive symptoms.[45] Moderation by clinical experts was crucial to the more successful social media-based interventions.[45] Participants' who were less likely to actively engage in the intervention had more offline support or were shy.[45] This suggests face-to-face interventions play a different but valuable role and could complement offline interventions. Regarding interventions based on mobile applications (apps), only 23% of 121 apps marketed to treat anxiety utilized 2 or more evidence-based treatment modalities.[46] Another review assessing 15 mental health apps found no evidence that they help with teen mental health issues because they were marketed to do.[47] Recognizing the need to be

**Table 4**
**A Suggested Model to Clinically Evaluate Social Media Use Based on the "PQRST" Pain Model**

| Provoking Factors | Quality | Region/Radiation | Severity | Timing |
|---|---|---|---|---|
| Comorbid mental or physical health conditions | Style of SM use | How do you experience social media use physically? Mentally? | How is SM use getting in the way of functioning in different domains? | Frequency of use |
| | Type of SM use | | | Total time of use |
| Susceptibility to FOMO, peer-pressure, rejection sensitivity | Purpose of SM use | | Rate how problematic SM use is for you on a scale of 1 to 10 | Setting of use |
| | Platform(s) used | | | Time of day of use |
| Personality traits | Number of platforms used | | Incorporate validated assessment tools | Does anything influence use patterns positively or negatively? |

*Abbreviations:* FOMO–fear of missing out, SM–social media.
A suggested model to clinically evaluate social media use based on the "PQRST" pain evaluation model.

able to evaluate these apps, the Agency for Healthcare Research and Quality has developed the Framework to Assist Stakeholders in Technology Evaluation for Recovery to Mental Health and Wellness to guide consumers[48] and the American Psychiatric Association developed the publicly available "App Evaluation Model."[49]

## AS A FIELD, HOW DO WE HARNESS THE POWER OF SOCIAL MEDIA AS A PUBLIC MENTAL HEALTH TOOL?

Social media public health campaigns have successfully addressed autism awareness, tobacco cessation, and sexually transmitted infection screening, among other issues.[50] There were positive and negative associations related to COVID-19 provaccination versus antivaccination social media content and intent to vaccinate college students.[51] Clinicians can carry the successful social media-based public health principles into public mental health to scale our impact exponentially. National organizations should capitalize on social media's reach and influence with high quality, evidence-based curated content toward antistigma, psychoeducation, screening, and even intervention goals. Studies examining social media platforms as a potential screening tool for mental health issues have primarily focused on depression and suicide risk with limited but promising findings.[16] Innovative mental health providers are already using social media as a public health tool,[52] and social media platforms are implementing methods of verifying health-care providers to combat disinformation.[53] More researches are needed on how best to utilize social media as a public mental health tool, and we need to adapt the clinical and public health lessons we learn now to social media platforms because they rapidly evolve.

## CLINICS CARE POINTS

- Social media use and proposed related disorders are currently poorly defined and poorly operationalized.
- Social media use may positively or negatively influence the development throughout the life span, specifically during adolescence.
- Impacts of social media use have potential neurobiological correlates throughout development.
- There are weak correlational associations between anxiety and social media use in youth.
- Having and engaging in multiple social media accounts can indicate a higher risk of anxiety.
- There are many potential mediating and moderating variables, including FOMO, of social media use and anxiety.
- Parental monitoring of social media use may mitigate potential negative impacts.
- Assess social media use with a comprehensive clinical interview and validated assessment tools, although current assessment tools need updating.
- Treat underlying/comorbid psychiatric and physical ailments.
- Data on psychopharmacology to address problematic social media use are lacking.
- Data on therapy modalities are mixed but consider therapy with the specific goal of addressing problematic social media use by reinforcing other adaptive skills.
- Consider limiting social media use when it poses problems and incorporating social media use into a behavioral reward system.

- Develop ways to use social media as a public mental health tool through collaboration with national organizations.

## DECLARATION OF INTERESTS

Dr Croarkin has received research support from the Brain and Behavior Research Foundation, United States, Mayo Clinic Foundation, United States, National Institute of Mental Health, United States, National Science Foundation, Pfizer, United States, Neuronetics Inc., and NeoSync, United States. He has received equipment support from Neuronetics Inc. and MagVenture, United States for investigator-initiated research. He has received material support from Myriad Genetics, United States for investigator-initiated research. He has consulted for Engrail Therapeutics, Myriad Genetics, Procter & Gamble Company, and Sunovion.

## REFERENCES

1. Obar J, Wildman S. Social media definition and the governance challenge: an introduction to the special issue. SSRN Electron J 2015. https://doi.org/10.2139/ssrn.2637879.
2. Weinstein E. The social media see-saw: positive and negative influences on adolescents' affective well-being. New Media Soc 2018;20(10):3597–623.
3. Burke M, Kraut RE. The relationship between facebook use and well-being depends on communication type and tie strength. J Computer-Mediated Commun 2016;21(4):265–81.
4. Hancock J, Liu SX, Luo M, et al. Psychological well-being and social media use: a meta-analysis of associations between social media use and depression, anxiety, loneliness, eudaimonic, hedonic and social well-being. SSRN Electron J 2022. https://doi.org/10.2139/ssrn.4053961.
5. Vogels EA, Gelles-Watnick R, Massarat N. Teens, social media and technology 2022. Pew research center: internet, science & tech. Available at: https://www.pewresearch.org/internet/2022/08/10/teens-social-media-and-technology-2022/. Accessed November 11, 2022.
6. Glover J, Ariefdjohan M, Fritsch SL. KidsAnxiety and the digital world. Child Adolesc Psychiatr Clin N Am 2022;31(1):71–90. https://doi.org/10.1016/j.chc.2021.06.004.
7. NSCH datasets. United States census bureau. Available at: https://www.census.gov/programs-surveys/nsch/data/datasets.html. Accessed October 29, 2022.
8. Garnett MF, Curtin SC, Stone DM. Suicide mortality in the United States, 2000-2020. NCHS Data Brief 2022;(433):1–8.
9. Share of US households using specific technologies, 2005-2019. Our World in Data. Available at: https://ourworldindata.org/grapher/technology-adoption-by-households-in-the-united-states?time=2005..2019&country=~Social+media+usage. Accessed October 29, 2022.
10. Rideout V, Peebles A, Mann S. et al. Common Sense census: media use by tweens and teens, 2021, Available at: https://www.commonsensemedia.org/sites/default/files/research/report/8-18-census-integrated-report-final-web_0.pdf, Accessed October 29, 2022.
11. Bányai F, Zsila Á, Király O, et al. Problematic social media use: results from a large-scale nationally representative adolescent sample. PLoS One 2017;12(1):e0169839.

12. Müller SM, Wegmann E, Oelker A, et al. Assessment of Criteria for Specific Internet-use Disorders (ACSID-11): introduction of a new screening instrument capturing ICD-11 criteria for gaming disorder and other potential Internet-use disorders. Journal of Behavioral Addictions 2022 2022;11(2):427–50.

13. Orben A, Przybylski AK, Blakemore SJ, et al. Windows of developmental sensitivity to social media. Nat Commun 2022;13(1):1649.

14. Towner E, Grint J, Levy T, et al. Revealing the self in a digital world: a systematic review of adolescent online and offline self-disclosure. Curr Opin Psychol 2022; 45:101309.

15. Guinta MR. Social media and adolescent health, Pediatr Nurs, 2018;44(4): 196-201.

16. Primack BA, Perryman KL, Crofford RA, et al. Social media as it interfaces with psychosocial development and mental illness in transitional-age youth. Child Adolesc Psychiatr Clin N Am 2022;31(1):11–30.

17. Olvera C, Stebbins GT, Goetz CG, et al. TikTok tics: a pandemic within a pandemic. Mov Disord Clin Pract 2021;8(8):1200–5.

18. Arendt F, Scherr S, Romer D. Effects of exposure to self-harm on social media: evidence from a two-wave panel study among young adults. New Media Soc 2019;21(11–12):2422–42.

19. Sherman LE, Payton AA, Hernandez LM, et al. The power of the like in adolescence:effects of peer influence on neural and behavioral responses to social media. Psychol Sci 2016;27(7):1027–35.

20. Crone EA, Konijn EA. Media use and brain development during adolescence. Nat Commun 2018;9(1):588.

21. Steele RG, Hall JA, Christofferson JL. Conceptualizing digital stress in adolescents and young adults: toward the development of an empirically based model. Clin Child Fam Psychol Rev 2020;23(1):15–26.

22. Sherman LE, Hernandez LM, Greenfield PM, et al. What the brain 'Likes': neural correlates of providing feedback on social media. Soc Cognit Affect Neurosci 2018;13(7):699–707.

23. Stieger S, Wunderl S. Associations between social media use and cognitive abilities: results from a large-scale study of adolescents. Comput Human Behav 2022;135:107358.

24. Shannon H, Bush K, Villeneuve PJ, et al. Problematic social media use in adolescents and young adults: systematic review and meta-analysis. JMIR Ment Health 2022;9(4):e33450.

25. Hökby S, Hadlaczky G, Westerlund J, et al. Are mental health effects of internet use attributable to the web-based content or perceived consequences of usage? A longitudinal study of european adolescents. JMIR Ment Health 2016;3(3):e31.

26. Alonzo R, Hussain J, Stranges S, et al. Interplay between social media use, sleep quality, and mental health in youth: a systematic review. Sleep Med Rev 2021;56: 101414.

27. Piteo EM, Ward K. Review: social networking sites and associations with depressive and anxiety symptoms in children and adolescents - a systematic review. Child Adolesc Ment Health 2020;25(4):201–16.

28. Cataldo I, Lepri B, Neoh MJY, et al. Social media usage and development of psychiatric disorders in childhood and adolescence: a review. Front Psychiatry 2020; 11:508595.

29. Marino C, Gini G, Vieno A, et al. The associations between problematic Facebook use, psychological distress and well-being among adolescents and young adults: a systematic review and meta-analysis. J Affect Disord 2018;226:274–81.

30. Hussain Z, Griffiths MD. Problematic social networking site use and comorbid psychiatric disorders: a systematic review of recent large-scale studies. Front Psychiatry 2018;9:686.

31. Mougharbel F, Goldfield GS. Psychological correlates of sedentary screen time behaviour among children and adolescents: a narrative review. Curr Obes Rep 2020;9(4):493–511.

32. Ghaemi SN. Digital depression: a new disease of the millennium? Acta Psychiatr Scand 2020;141(4):356–61.

33. Beyens I, Keijsers L, Coyne SM. Social media, parenting, and well-being. Curr Opin Psychol 2022;47:101350.

34. Odgers CL, Jensen MR. Annual research review: adolescent mental health in the digital age: facts, fears, and future directions. J Child Psychol Psychiatry 2020; 61(3):336–48.

35. Sarmiento IG, Olson C, Yeo G, et al. How does social media use relate to adolescents' internalizing symptoms? Conclusions from a systematic narrative review. Adolescent Research Review 2020;5(4):381–404.

36. Kovačić Petrović Z, Peraica T, Kozarić-Kovačić D, et al. Internet use and internet-based addictive behaviours during coronavirus pandemic. Curr Opin Psychiatry 2022;35(5):324–31.

37. Haddad JM, Macenski C, Mosier-Mills A, et al. The impact of social media on college mental health during the COVID-19 pandemic: a multinational review of the existing literature. Curr Psychiatry Rep 2021;23(11):70.

38. Zdanowicz N, Reynaert C, Jacques D, et al. Screen time and (Belgian) teenagers. Psychiatr Danub 2020;32(Suppl 1):36–41.

39. Twenge JM, Joiner TE, Rogers ML, et al. Increases in depressive symptoms, suicide-related outcomes, and suicide rates among US adolescents after 2010 and links to increased new media screen time. Clin Psychol Sci 2018;6(1):3–17.

40. Hutson E, Kelly S, Militello LK. Systematic review of cyberbullying interventions for youth and parents with implications for evidence-based practice. Worldviews Evid Based Nurs 2018;15(1):72–9.

41. Lupton D. Young people's use of digital health technologies in the global north: narrative review. J Med Internet Res 2021;23(1):e18286.

42. Nereim C, Bickham D, Rich M. A primary care pediatrician's guide to assessing problematic interactive media use. Curr Opin Pediatr 2019;31(4):435–41.

43. Cataldo I, Billieux J, Esposito G, et al. Assessing problematic use of social media: where do we stand and what can be improved? Current Opinion in Behavioral Sciences 2022;45:101145.

44. Hill DL. Social media: anticipatory guidance. Pediatr Rev 2020;41(3):112–9.

45. Ridout B, Campbell A. The use of social networking sites in mental health interventions for young people: systematic review. J Med Internet Res 2018;20(12): e12244.

46. Bry LJ, Chou T, Miguel E, et al. Consumer smartphone apps marketed for child and adolescent anxiety: a systematic review and content analysis. Behav Ther 2018;49(2):249–61.

47. Grist R, Porter J, Stallard P. Mental health mobile apps for preadolescents and adolescents: a systematic review. J Med Internet Res 2017;19(5):e176.

48. Agarwal S, Jalan M, Wilcox HC, et al. AHRQ comparative effectiveness technical briefs. evaluation of mental health mobile applications. Rockville, MD: Agency for Healthcare Research and Quality (US; 2022.

49. The app evaluation model. American psychiatric association. Available at: https://www.psychiatry.org/psychiatrists/practice/mental-health-apps/the-app-evaluation-model. Accessed October 29, 2022.

50. Pinto R, Silva L, Valentim R, et al. Systematic review on information technology approaches to evaluate the impact of public health campaigns: real cases and possible directions. Front Public Health 2021;9:715403.

51. Luo S, Xin M, Wang S, et al. Behavioural intention of receiving COVID-19 vaccination, social media exposures and peer discussions in China. Epidemiol Infect 2021;149:1–33.

52. Sobowale K, Kaliebe K. Appealing applications for adolescent mental health: social media's transformation during the COVID-19 pandemic. J Am Acad Child Adolesc Psychiatry 2021;60(10):S4.

53. Diaz N. YouTube to extend verified healthcare source status to individual providers. Becker's Healthcare. Available at: https://www.beckershospitalreview.com/digital-marketing/youtube-to-extend-verified-healthcare-source-status-to-individual-providers.html. Accessed October 29, 2022.

# All Shades of Anxiety

## A Review of Therapeutic and Psychotropic Considerations for Child and Adolescent Youth of Color

Michele Cosby, PsyD, LCP[a],[*],[1], Dimal D. Shah, MD[a],[1],
Stella Lopez, PsyD, LCP[b],[1], Jlynn Holland-Cecil, MS[c],[2],
Michael Keiter, BS[d],[3], Crystal Lewis, BS[d],[4],
Cheryl S. Al-Mateen, MD, DFAPA[a],[e],[1]

## KEYWORDS

- Anxiety • BIPOC • Implicit bias • Inequities • Intersectionality • Youth of color

## KEY POINTS

- Black, Indigenous, and other persons of color (BIPOC) youth with anxiety experience an additional impact specifically related to social differences, disparities, and inequities in access to care as well as individual, familial, and systemic barriers to adequate care.
- These differences, disparities, and inequities occur at national, community, familial, and individual levels.
- Ongoing clinician education regarding the impact of culture on clinical presentation and interventions for BIPOC youth will allow us to increase accurate treatment and support for this population.

## INTRODUCTION

There is a significant body of research focused on risk factors for anxiety disorders. It is essential to also highlight the factors that contribute to and exacerbate the presentation and treatment of anxiety in youth of color (**Boxes 1–4**). Youth who identify as

[a] Department of Psychiatry, Virginia Commonwealth University, PO Box 980489, Richmond, VA 23220, USA; [b] Virginia Treatment Center for Children VCU Health, Richmond, VA, USA; [c] Virginia State University, Petersburg, VA, USA; [d] Virginia Commonwealth University, Richmond, VA, USA; [e] Department of Pediatrics, Virginia Commonwealth University, Richmond, VA, USA
[1] Present address: PO Box 980489, Richmond, VA 23220.
[2] Present address: 3707 Morgan Trail Drive, Chesterfield, VA, 23832.
[3] Present address: 1235 Prosperity Road, Virginia Beach, VA 23451.
[4] Present address: 1205 Redwood Valley Lane, Knightdale, NC 27545.
* Corresponding author.
*E-mail address:* Michele.cosby@vcuhealth.org

Child Adolesc Psychiatric Clin N Am 32 (2023) 631–653
https://doi.org/10.1016/j.chc.2023.02.007
1056-4993/23/© 2023 Elsevier Inc. All rights reserved.

> **Box 1**
> **Clinical case—Ruby (1)**
>
> Ruby is a 12-year-old Black bisexual girl who uses she/her pronouns who presents to the outpatient psychiatric clinic to establish care 5 days after being discharged from her first acute inpatient psychiatric hospitalization. Ruby was admitted for suicidal ideations with plan to overdose on over-the-counter medications found in the home or cut herself with a "sharp knife." Ruby had been feeling significantly overwhelmed by her worsening intrusive thoughts during the 7 months. These thoughts caused sleep latency of approximately 2 hours each night. She had nightmares most nights and had difficulty falling back to sleep. She ruminated about recent interactions with peers at school, her future, her mother's health, her school performance, and potentially doing something embarrassing in front of her peers. She did not like to be called on or asked to talk aloud in class. She frequently avoided social engagements and school. Ruby missed 15 days of the past 45 days of school. In the morning, she would oversleep and miss the school bus, complain of severe stomach aches, or barter with her mother to allow her to stay home. Ruby identified herself as a "worry-wart" and a perfectionist. She preferred routine and structure throughout her day. She became more anxious with unpredictable alterations from her routine. During her anxious "episodes," she engaged in catastrophic thinking and all-or-none thinking, as well as experienced palpitations, gastrointestinal distress, globus pharyngeus, depersonalization, and derealization. She denied panic attacks or fear of future ones.
>
> During the evaluation, Ruby sat in the chair holding an old, grungy plush doll with both hands and rested on her stomach. She clutched it tighter when discussing her anxiety symptoms and current stressors. Patient was constricted, anxious, guarded, and selectively mute throughout the interview. She preferred her mother answer most, if not all, questions, which the mother did until Ruby was interviewed individually. Although Ruby was hospitalized, her mother secured the home of dangerous items and locked up all medications in the home. Ruby had not engaged in self-injurious or suicidal behaviors since discharge from the hospital.

Black, Indigenous, or persons of color (BIPOC) experience developmental stressors that affect school, peer relationships, relationships with family, and in the community. The addition of race-related stress can also serve to increase risk factors for this population. For the purposes of this review, we use Black and Latinx to be inclusive of the multiple races, ethnicities, and gender identities of these populations.

> **Box 2**
> **Clinical case—Ruby (2)**
>
> Ruby had no previous psychiatric history except for her first and only acute inpatient psychiatric hospitalization. She had not attempted suicide or engaged in nonsuicidal self-injurious behaviors since hospitalization. Ruby did not have any allergies to medications and denied ever using any substances. Her pertinent medical history included morbid obesity, visible keloids with hyperpigmented healed scars on her arms and neck, polycystic ovarian syndrome, and prediabetes mellitus, which is managed by a local pediatric endocrinologist. She had no past surgical history.
>
> She lived in a modest home with her single mother, who had shared custody with her father whom she visited some weekends. She had her own room, where she frequently retreated throughout the day. Her paternal family identified as Baptist while her maternal family was less religious. She identified as a Black bisexual girl who is not sexually active. She has had one boyfriend and one girlfriend in the past. She has disclosed her sexuality to her mother, who was accepting. She attended sixth grade at a public middle school. She earned mostly Bs. She previously had a 504 plan to provide accommodations for her anxiety symptoms. School administrators encouraged Ruby and her mother to seek homebound alternative at-home online schooling because Ruby missed 15 days of school during the past 45 days.

Box 3
Clinical case—diagnosis for Ruby (3)

|  | Differential Diagnosis | Final Diagnosis |
|---|---|---|
| Psychiatric | Generalized anxiety disorder | Generalized anxiety disorder |
|  | Social anxiety disorder | Social anxiety disorder |
|  | Separation anxiety disorder |  |
|  | Specific phobia |  |
|  | Agoraphobia |  |
|  | Attention deficit hyperactivity disorder |  |
|  | Adjustment disorder with anxious distress |  |
|  | Posttraumatic stress disorder |  |
|  | Schizophrenia |  |
|  | Dissociative identity disorder |  |
| Nonpsychiatric | Cardiac conditions | Polycystic ovarian syndrome |
|  | Substances (inhalants, cannabis, stimulants) | Keloids |
|  | Seizures (temporal lobe or herpes simplex virus) | Morbid obesity prediabetes mellitus |
|  | Malingering |  |
|  | Malignancies (brain mass) |  |
|  | Meningitis, encephalitis |  |

Crenshaw[1] coined the term "intersectionality" to highlight the unique and interrelated experiences of an individual's marginalized identities/perceptions rather than as independently linked (ie, being Black and transgender). Intersectionality blends these perspectives and explains their idiosyncratic ties and clarifies how each identity is interwoven.[2] The framework also attends to how US society functions by dominant culture (White, male, middle-class and up, heterosexual, cis-gendered, able-bodied, college-educated, and so forth) and explains how oppression, prejudice, and discrimination affect each marginalized identity, thus limiting access to power and privilege. Overwhelming research finds cumulative discrimination exacerbates negative mental health outcomes (such as psychological distress, depressive, and anxiety-related symptoms) across underserved communities, especially for those with intersectional identities.

Box 4
Clinical case: treatment recommendations and outcomes for Ruby (4)

Recommendations:
- Med Management:
  ○ Sertraline initiated at 25 mg nightly and titrated to an effective dose of 125 mg nightly
  ○ Hydroxyzine 25 mg 3 times per day as needed for acute anxiety
- Psychotherapeutic:
  ○ Cognitive behavioral therapy with a trauma-informed lens.
  ○ Parent Management: Psychoeducation and review of coping strategies
  ○ Dialectical behavioral therapy group for parent and child
  ○ Postacute hospitalization referred for in-home intensive therapy for additional stabilization

Outcomes:
Ruby identified reduction in worry and perfectionistic tendencies as well as increased range of tolerance for discomfort. She did not have any new incidents of self-injurious behavior and denied any active suicidal ideation with fleeting passive suicidal thoughts occurring once when at her father's house. Otherwise, Ruby utilized a safety plan of checking in with mother when noticing an increase in worry. She discussed plans of returning to in-person education this academic year in partnership with her local public school counseling team

This is especially important to conceptualize when including lesbian, gay, bisexual, transgender, questioning, queer, intersex, asexual, and pansexual (LGBTQIA+) identities due to the different layers of discrimination both within their racial group (sexism, homophobia, and transphobia) and outside (racism, sexism, homophobia, and transphobia). An increase in health disparities and worse health outcomes is likely to be exacerbated for youth with multiple minority status identities.[3] Mental health stigma is present and known; there are limited studies addressing the impacts of intersectionality on mental illness.[4] Because identity development is significantly critical during adolescence, it is important to understand the impact of behaviors and attitudes on mental illness/treatment-seeking stigma.[4] It is commonly understood that anxiety is much more prevalent among women, although not as much research is available on individuals holding transgender female identities.[5]

Youth of color experience a layer of racial stigma and a second label of mental health stigma, which may lead to limited reports of their psychological disturbances. They are less likely to process their mental health with peers, may experience poor responses from peers for seeking services, and also experience increased self-stigma and public stigma from family and peers comparatively to their White peers.[4,6–9]

## PREVALENCE AND INCIDENCE

According to the National Comorbidity Survey: Adolescent Supplement, anxiety disorders are the most common mental health diagnosis in the adolescent population, affecting 1 in 3 adolescents on average in the United States.[10] The average age of onset for mental health disorders was the earliest for anxiety relative to other conditions, starting at 6 years of age (11 years of age for behavioral disorders, 13 years of age for mood disorders, and 15 years of age for substance use disorders).[10] The national prevalence of youth with a mental illness is steadily increasing but the "need" for mental health services far outweighs the "supply" (and reach) of mental health providers in this country. BIPOC youth have some of the most alarming rates of unmet mental health needs—in the context of anxiety.

There are trends in the prevalence, severity, and identification of anxiety disorders across different racial/ethnic groups. When assessing anxiety disorders in Black youth, multiple studies have shown that Black children and adolescents meet criteria for an anxiety disorder at a significantly higher rate than White children and adolescents in the United States.[10,11] Studies also show a steeper rate of increase in anxiety disorders across multiple generations (grouped by cohorts based on birth year from 1957 to 1969, 1970 to 1982, and 1983 to 1991) for Black Americans compared with White Americans, with Black youth having almost double the prevalence of anxiety disorders compared with White youth today.[11] Research regarding racial differences in the prevalence of specific subtypes of anxiety disorders is scarce, however, some studies suggest that Black children may have higher rates of simple phobia, posttraumatic stress disorder, and obsessive compulsive disorder compared with their White counterparts.[12,13] One study also found that White children with anxiety were more likely to present to clinics with school refusal to attend and have higher clinician-reported severity ratings than Black children.[12] The perception of more severe anxiety in White children was most likely confounded by the fact that all clinician interviewers and researchers in the study were White. Findings hypothesized that racial bias was involved and that White providers reported an increased clinician-rated severity of anxiety symptoms of White youth compared with Black youth. The reasoning behind why White children may have had higher rates of school refusal is unclear.[12] There are overall gaps in the literature regarding differences in severity of anxiety in Black youth compared with other racial groups. However, this particular finding brings forth the question of how clinician biases may play a role in how childhood mental health disorders are perceived, diagnosed, and subsequently treated in the United States. Diagnostic biases that tend to focus on more externalizing symptoms in youth of color rather than more internalizing experiences of anxiety can lead to ineffective treatment and increase in symptom severity if anxiety disorders are not identified and diagnosed appropriately.

As for Latinx youth, multiple studies have noted significantly higher rates of separation anxiety and worry compared with other racial/ethnic groups.[14–16] Some also quote higher rates of global anxiety, physical symptoms of anxiety, and psychiatric comorbidities specifically in Latinx women.[16] Another trend worthy of noting is the decreased rate of symptom identification in Latinx youth with anxiety.[15,17] Compared with White parents, Mexican and Mexican American parents were more likely to interpret relatively ambiguous symptoms (ie, "On the way to school you begin to feel funny in your stomach") as nonpsychiatric in nature as opposed to somatic symptoms related to anxiety.[15] The research team hypothesized this may be due to a culturally decreased likelihood to interpret such symptoms as being psychiatric in nature. The authors encourage clinicians to be aware of this interpretation bias to minimize misdiagnosis.[15] Similarly, Tarshis, Jutte, and Huffman[17] found that pediatricians had more difficulty identifying internalizing disorders in low-socioeconomic status Latinx youth compared with other mental health problems. As we know, systemically, the discord between the amount of information primary care providers are ideally expected to obtain with each visit and the amount of time allotted makes covering topics such as mental health much more difficult. However, the lack of these critical conversations for all children may leave youth potentially in need of mental health services both underdiagnosed and undertreated. The routine use of screening instruments either before or during appointments may be helpful in this regard (**Table 1** for examples of screening instruments).

Aside from Black and Latinx youth, research on the prevalence or manifestations of anxiety disorders in youth from other racial/ethnic minority groups is severely lacking. Some of the literature points toward American Indian/Alaskan Native adolescents as having significantly higher rates of anxiety and depression than White adolescents; however, this report was specifically within the context of children with special health care needs (ie, asthma, diabetes).[18] Another study involving Asian American and "Other" racial minorities, in addition to Black and Latinx youth, found that all 4 of these racial minority groups reported more severe anxiety symptoms and more frequently lived in disadvantaged neighborhoods than Whites. There was also an additive relationship between these 2 variables, with children belonging to both a racial minority group and disadvantaged neighborhood tending to have the most severe anxiety symptoms of all the groups.[19] It is our obligation as health professionals to turn our lens toward BIPOC youth as a particularly high-risk but often overlooked group of individuals worthy of more focus in this area (**Table 2** for cultural aspects of Anxiety in DSM-5-TR).

Adverse childhood experiences (ACEs) are negative and potentially traumatic events such as abuse, neglect, and household dysfunction that occur before the age of 18 years.[27] When assessing the impact of ACEs on childhood mental health, studies have shown that ACE scores are a significant and dose-dependent predictor of anxiety, depression, and behavioral/conduct problems in youth aged 3 to 17 years.[28] It is important to note that certain racial/ethnic groups, especially Black and Latinx youth, are most often exposed to higher amounts of ACEs than other racial groups and thus are at higher risk of mental health disorders.[29] Racial disparities also

**Table 1**
Anxiety screeners

| Scale | Parent Version | Child Version | Age Range (y) | Conducted by Clinician? | Length (min) | Cost? | Resource |
|---|---|---|---|---|---|---|---|
| SCARED | Yes | Yes | 8–18 | No | ~10 min | Free | https://www.pediatricbipolar.pitt.edu/resources/instruments |
| Generalized anxiety disorder-7 | No | Yes | 12+ | No | ~5 min | Free | https://www.apaservices.org/practice/measurement-based-care/suggested-measures |
| GADSS-Child | No | Yes | 11–17 | No | ~5 min | Free | https://www.psychiatry.org/File%20Library/Psychiatrists/Practice/DSM/APA_DSM5_Severity-Measure-For-Generalized-Anxiety-Disorder-Child-Age-11-to-17.pdf |
| Beck Anxiety Inventory | No | Yes | 12+ | No | ~10 min | Free | https://www.apaservices.org/practice/measurement-based-care/suggested-measures |
| Preschool Anxiety Scale | Yes | No | 2.5–6.5 | Yes | ~20 min | Free | https://www.scaswebsite.com/ |
| Spence Child Anxiety Scale | Yes | Yes | 8–15 | Yes | ~15 min | Free | https://www.scaswebsite.com/ |
| Hamilton Anxiety Rating Scale | No | Yes | All? | Yes | ~15 min | Free | https://psychology-tools.com/test/hamilton-anxiety-rating-scale |

| Table 2 |
|---|
| **Cultural features of diagnostic and statistical manual of mental disorders diagnoses** |

| DSM Diagnosis: | Clinical Correlates: |
|---|---|
| Generalized anxiety disorder | • Some cultures show more somatic symptoms, and others have more cognitive symptoms<br>• Social and cultural contexts are critical in evaluating if worries about situations are excessive[20,21]<br>• In the United States, higher rates are associated with racism/ethnic discrimination<br>• Higher income countries meet diagnostic criteria more often than lower income countries |
| Social anxiety disorder | • US non-Latinx Whites have an earlier age of onset compared with US Latinx even though Latinx have greater impairments<br>• Immigrant status is associated with lower rates in White groups (Latinx and non-Latinx)[20]<br>• *Taijin kyofusho* is a syndrome seen in Japan and Korea, which can meet criteria for social anxiety disorder, body dysmorphic disorder or delusional disorder |
| Separation anxiety disorder | • Cultural variation based on individual subgroups: What level of separation is desirable for the culture? When is it appropriate to leave the parental home? |
| Selective mutism | • Individuals who need to speak in a nonnative language (children of immigrant families) have a higher risk of developing this disorder[22]<br>• Children who have immigrated to a country with a different language may *appear* to have this if they refuse to speak the new language because of lack of knowledge |
| Specific phobia | • Lower prevalence is seen in persons of Asian and Latinx descent than in Non-Latinx Whites and African Americans[23] |
| Panic disorder | • Cultural expectations may influence whether panic attacks are expected or unexpected[20]<br>• Cultural concepts of distress associated with panic disorder include *ataque de nervios* in Latin Americans and *khyâl* (wind attacks) in Cambodians[20]<br>• Culture specific symptoms of panic "may include tinnitus, neck soreness, headache, and uncontrollable screaming or crying[24] (P. 244)<br>• Higher rates of paresthesias may be seen in African Americans<br>• Higher rates of dizziness may be seen in several Asian groups, that is, *khyâl* (wind attacks) in Cambodians, which includes dizziness, tinnitus, and neck soreness<br>• Higher rates of trembling may be seen in non-Latinx Whites<br>• *Ataque de nervios* (attack of nerves) is a cultural syndrome in Latin Americans that may include trembling, uncontrollable screaming or crying, aggressive or suicidal behavior, and depersonalization or derealization[20]<br>• Panic disorder is associated with reports of racism and ethnic discrimination in Asian Americans, Hispanic Americans and African Americans in the United States[25]<br>• The rate of help-seeking (use of mental health services) varies across ethnic and racial groups[26] for panic disorder<br>• There is less impairment in samples of non-Latinx whites than African Americans in the United States[20] |

(continued on next page)

| Table 2 (continued) | |
|---|---|
| **DSM Diagnosis:** | **Clinical Correlates:** |
| | • Lower prevalence estimates are found in Latinx/African Americans/Caribbean Blacks/Asian Americans when compared with non-Latinx Whites. However, in American Indian populations, panic disorder ranges from 2.6% to 4.1%[20] |
| Agoraphobia | • DSM does not specifically mention differences among cultures |

Note all information collected from DSM-5-TR. [American Psychiatric Association. (2022). Diagnostic and Statistical Manual of Mental Disorders (5th ed., text rev.). [https://doi.org/10.1176/appi.books.9780890425787].

exist within mental health diagnoses of children exposed to ACEs, with Black children being 1.2 times more likely than White or Latinx children to be diagnosed with behavioral/conduct disorders as opposed to internalizing disorders such as anxiety or depression.[28] Conversely, White children exposed to ACEs were 1.77 times more likely to be diagnosed with depression and 2.61 times more likely to be diagnosed with anxiety compared with Black children.[28] These racial mental health diagnostic disparities raise concern that minoritized youth may be misdiagnosed and/or underdiagnosed regarding trauma-related internalizing and externalizing disorders and thus are at risk of not receiving the treatment or resources that they need.

## ADDITIONAL CONSIDERATIONS
### Racism and Race-Related Stress

When caring for BIPOC youth with anxiety, it is imperative to consider the impact that racism and discrimination can have on one's experience. Unsurprisingly, children and adolescents who experience racial discrimination are at a much higher risk of developing anxiety, depression, and a host of other nonpsychiatric health conditions, compared with the general public.[30] In fact, higher levels of racism-related stress are directly correlated with higher levels of anxiety.[30] Frequent online and social media coverage of race-based violence or injustice can also significantly affect the mental health of BIPOC youth. Although these platforms help to increase awareness of these events, they have also been found to evoke trauma-related symptoms and increase anxiety in youth of color.[31]

Many downstream effects of systemic racism and oppression also contribute to the racial disparities seen in socioeconomic status, education, and health care in a plethora of ways. In the realm of mental health, many minoritized individuals living in lower socioeconomic communities are forced to prioritize their basic needs over their mental health or, similarly, lack the insurance or financial means required to participate in mental health care.[32] Furthermore, many underserved communities are associated with higher incidence of violence or trauma, which places minoritized youth in those communities at an even higher risk for both anxiety and depression.[32] Whether through direct exposure to racial discrimination or through indirect disadvantages imposed on them by racialized systemic practices, this leaves the mental health of our BIPOC youth in a particularly vulnerable place.

### Impact of COVID-19

The identification of stressors within these communities provides the opportunity to identify key protective factors to benefit BIPOC adolescent mental health and prevent the development of anxiety disorders. Family support serves as a protective factor due to the positive relationships within families. Families also serve to affect access to care. BIPOC adolescents may be denying the need for services as a means of protecting their caregivers from additional stress and strain within the family system.[33] COVID-19 significantly affected the entire population and was documented to disproportionately influence communities of color. The highest levels of racism experienced by BIPOC youth during the stay-at-home period of the pandemic were reported among Asian students (64%), Black students (55%), and students of multiple races (55%).[34]

Several experiences significantly increased anxiety within youth.[35] The existing barriers particularly for Black adolescents to utilize mental health services intensified during the pandemic.[35] Struggles during the peak of the pandemic included attending school from home, being separated from their peers, and the intensified impact on family hardships. As minority youth returned to a more normative school environment, they completed less school assignments, had an increase in screen time, and a more significant impact on their mental health overall.[35] Studies document that Black youth in particular experienced an increase in distress and financial concerns due to their own exposure to COVID-19 as well as family members contracting COVID.[33] The health disparities that led to the disproportionate death rate in many Black communities affected children and adolescents disproportionately as well. This was particularly significant in single-parent families. Furthermore, there was repetitive COVID-19 media coverage, increased use of social media, and the likelihood of having a family member providing direct care and on the front line.[33]

The actual impact of COVID-19 also fueled anxiety for black adolescents due to fear of leaving their homes. Therefore, it is imperative that we recognize and understand the benefits and the necessity of maintaining access to telehealth to relieve anxiety in this particular population moving forward.[33] The pandemic also highlighted the intersection between the pandemic and social determinants as well as their influence on youth of color. A syndemic is "the synergistic nature of the health and social problems facing the poor and underserved.[36]"(pg. 225). In this context, we refer to the junction of COVID-19 and systemic racism highlighted by the impact of the pandemic, the killing of George Floyd, and additional occurrences of racial violence, which inevitably magnified uncertainty for youth of color. The Mott Poll Report in 2020 highlighted the top health concerns for kids during the pandemic, noting the differing priorities between racial/ethnic groups. The report noted that for Black parents, the top 2 child concerns were racism and COVID-19, whereas both Hispanic and White parents top 2 child concerns included overuse of social media and bullying/cyberbullying. The complete report can be found at: https://mottpoll.org/reports/top-health-concerns-kids-2020-during-pandemic. The frequency and increased visibility hate crimes against many populations of color including Black and Asian individuals, elevated the experience of anxiety in BIPOC youth and their families.[37,38]

Within the Latinx community, interesting findings were collected by researchers that demonstrated distinct findings from the Black community in that COVID-19 social restrictions may have been beneficial to Latinx youth.[39] Several factors were suggested to have beneficial effects on this population's mental health including increased time with family, removal from potentially negative school or peer interactions, and more autonomy within youth academic schedules.[39] However, these findings were not found to be universal within the Latinx/Hispanic community. Roche and colleagues[40] determined that an increase in an adolescent's childcare responsibilities occurred in response to several factors to include parental figures or family being hospitalized, working, or job loss within the home during the COVID-19 pandemic. These responsibilities had a negative influence on both their mental health and GPA of these youth.

Although there were negative influences, the increase in family connection also served as a protective against stress. This is suggestive that mental health decline and increased stress is related to more parental-type responsibility and decrease in availability of time for studies. The increase in family connectivity, thought protective from mental health concerns for some youth, also provided increased responsibility and likelihood of increased stressors.

The Asian American/Pacific Islander (AAPI) community, although not new to feeling the intensive and negative effects of racism and discrimination, had more visibility in this regard during the COVID-19 pandemic. The increased prevalence in media coverage provided an additional source of stress for youth and adults within the AAPI community,[37] while additionally experiencing targeted physical and emotional abuse. Specifically within the AAPI community in the height of the COVID-19 pandemic, racism and discrimination were key sources of poor academic performance, mental health decline, and the development of anxiety within adolescent youth.[34]

LGBTQ + youth with intersectional identities related to also being BIPOC, of low socioeconomic status, or those experiencing homelessness also had an increased risk of anxiety during the pandemic. Only 33% of LGBTQ + youth lived in an affirming home during the pandemic. This may have increased the intensity of rejection or abuse by families and further separated them from supportive resources due to school shutdowns, remote learning, and social isolation. All of these things resulted in an increase in anxiety and depressive symptoms in this particular population.[41]

### Generational Anxiety

The prevalence of anxiety in childhood has steadily increased during the years across all racial/ethnic groups. Older generations report much lower rates of childhood-onset anxiety than children today.[11] However, racial differences exist in how the prevalence of childhood anxiety disorders has changed since the 1960s.[11] One study by Louie and Wheaton looked specifically at the Black–White patterning of mental disorders across different generations. They found that Black individuals in the oldest cohort (32–44 years old) had lower rates of anxiety disorders in childhood than their White counterparts.[11] Black individuals in the middle cohort (19–31 years old), however, showed no difference in the rate of anxiety disorders in childhood relative to White participants. Finally, Black participants in the youngest cohort (13–18 years old) showed higher rates of anxiety disorders than their White peers. In fact, Black adolescents in the youngest cohort had almost double the prevalence of anxiety than White adolescents (33.4% vs 16.3%, respectively). Furthermore, Black Americans showed a steeper rate of increase in anxiety disorders across generational cohorts compared with the rate observed for whites during the same period.[11] This increase in anxiety disorders in progressive generations is consistent with the burgeoning epigenetic/biology literature connecting maternal adverse childhood experiences to childhood psychopathology, including anxiety through the transmission of shortened telomeres.[42]

Other studies in the literature also highlight the trends in anxiety disorder prevalence relating to immigration generations and race/ethnicity. Of note, Latinx youth in these studies were more likely to come from low-income families; however, research that was inclusive of the impact of immigration status is lacking in the literature. Georgiades and colleagues[43] found that the first-generation (adolescents born outside of the United States) Black, Asian, and Latinx immigrant adolescents had higher odds of developing mood/anxiety disorders compared with the second-generation (adolescent born in the United States with both parents/single parent born in the United States) White immigrant adolescents. There was also an increased risk for the second-generation (adolescents born in the United States with at least one parent born outside of the United States) Black and Asian immigrant adolescents and third-generation Black and Latinx immigrant adolescents to develop a mood/anxiety disorder compared with the third-generation White immigrant adolescents.[43] Georgiades and colleagues also found that the first-generation Asian, White, and Latinx immigrants, along with first-generation, second-generation, and third-generation Black immigrants had a decreased use of mental health services as well. All of these generational trends highlighting the prevalence of youth with anxiety disorders point toward a common theme that, although all racial/ethnic groups are experiencing a shift toward increased prevalence of anxiety disorders, this relationship is even more pronounced for marginalized communities. The data also highlights first-generation minoritized immigrants as a group particularly at risk of having their mental health needs unmet.[43]

## DISPARITIES IN ACCESS AND CARE: SOCIAL DETERMINANTS OF MENTAL HEALTH

A study conducted by Brewer and colleagues[44] in Illinois found that, among 39,507 children aged 5 to 19 years who presented to the emergency department (ED) with a primary diagnosis of anxiety or depression, Latinx youth were significantly less likely to be hospitalized than their non-Latinx White peers. Non-Latinx Black youth were also less likely to be hospitalized than their White peers; however, this finding was not statistically significant. The study also found that children who were on Medicaid or uninsured were less likely to be hospitalized than children with private insurance, despite the groups presenting to the ED at similar frequencies.[44] Overall, the inability for BIPOC youth and their families to access mental health services due to their inability to financially afford or geographically locate a specialist within their communities, as well as receive equitable care despite various sociodemographic factors places these children at a much higher risk for poorer outcomes as a result of their unmet mental health needs.[44]

Various societal perceptions and social determinants heavily influence our ability to access and engage with mental health services. Marginalized communities often deal with these factors to a much greater extent, which is most likely why minoritized, low-income, and rural communities have some of the highest levels of unmet mental health needs.[32] Geographic location has been a significant barrier to individuals in underserved communities accessing mental health services due to the shortage of specialists in or near these communities. As a result, most minoritized individuals seek mental health care from ED or community centers instead of mental health specialists.[32,45] In fact, compared with White adolescents in the United States, American Indian/Alaskan Native, Black, and Latinx adolescents have significantly greater odds of experiencing difficulties obtaining specialty care.[46] Other commonly cited barriers to treatment include the elevated cost of mental health services, concerns regarding insurance coverage, and available/reliable transportation.[32,47] Several studies have identified racial/ethnic minority groups, specifically Black, Latinx, and American Indian/Alaskan Native, as having some of the highest rates of uninsured or publicly insured individuals in the United States.[32,46] Some studies also show that race and insurance coverage can even affect a child's likelihood of being psychiatrically hospitalized.[44]

### Parental Beliefs Regarding Treatment: Stigma and Alternative Coping

Parents are effectively the gatekeepers when it comes to children pursuing mental health treatment and what that treatment ultimately looks like. Therefore, it is important to recognize how parents' perceptions of mental health and treatment options affect whether a child is able to get the help that they need.

In addition to physical barriers, "attitudinal barriers" such as "denial, mistrust, or stigmatization of help-seeking" often prevent BIPOC youth from accessing mental health resources.[32] Racial/ethnic minorities' mistrust of the health-care system and predominantly White institutions stems from the centuries of oppression and exploitation imposed on minoritized communities. The exposure to racism and prejudice within the US health-care system and society has also heightened the level of mistrust that minority groups feel toward health-care professionals. When surveying a group of African American mothers in rural Georgia about their perceptions on seeking mental health help for their children, the single most frequently endorsed barrier to help-seeking was cultural mistrust, followed by stigma.[47] In fact, one-third of mothers thought that White providers would not be able to understand the problems of African American families, and 17% were concerned that White providers would not treat their Black children as well as they would treat a White child.[47] Furthermore, parental self-stigma, which involves one's own psychological distress, perceived discrimination, feeling othered, and perceived stigmatization by others for seeking help for mental health plays a large role.[48] For example, some studies report that almost 50% of black mothers worry that their community will find out that their child is seeing a mental health professional, and 16% were concerned about what others in the community would think/say about their child receiving help for emotional or behavioral problems.[47] Even Latinx and Black adolescents with a diagnosed mental illness have reported stigmatization from their own communities such as through family members rejecting the youth's diagnosis (ie, "you don't need to be taking no pills, cause you're not sick"), dissuading them from disclosing their diagnosis or seeking treatment, and fearing that disclosing their diagnosis would bring shame to them and their families.[8] As a result of stigma and cultural mistrust, many racial/ethnic minority groups also prefer to address mental health concerns on their own or to "keep things in the family," especially in Latinx or immigrant communities that may also fear deportation because of seeking help.[32] Therefore, provider–patient racial discordance, stigma, and cultural mistrust can play a significant role in whether BIPOC families feel comfortable engaging with and seeking help from mental health professionals. This also highlights how racial disparities in accessing mental health care are multifactorial and stem from a combination of systemic barriers as well as negative perceptions and stigmas regarding mental health in minoritized communities. Yusuf and colleagues propose that offering treatment services that engage family members and are culturally tailored could be potentially helpful at combating these disparities for BIPOC youth.[45]

The families of youth with anxiety disorders also experience significant burdens when it comes to the family's physical health, psychological well-being, and overall family functioning.[49] For BIPOC youth, the impact of mental health issues is often felt by the family unit.[50] Due to BIPOC families relying more heavily on familial resources in order to support other family members, this could likely contribute to an increase in accommodation behaviors for youth with anxiety disorders as a way to minimize external awareness of the intensity of anxiety symptoms.[49]

As for medication management, studies show that all parents, regardless of race, perceive antidepressants to be overall more effective but also riskier than psychotherapy for addressing child mental health issues.[51] Furthermore, parents who perceived greater benefits with antidepressant use were much more likely to follow-up at future medication visits[51]. Some of the biggest concerns from parents regarding antidepressant use were that their child would become addicted to the medication or cause suicidal urges.[51] Black parents overall perceived antidepressants to be both more risky and less beneficial than other racial groups, which could be a contributing factor as to why Black youth have lower rates of antidepressant use compared with White youth.[51]

### Spirituality-Supports Within Community

The preferred sources of support in communities of color for mental health challenges are typically communalistic or spiritually centered in nature to include family members, pastors/religious leaders, teachers, and school counselors.[47] Parents were asked: "Who would you most likely go to see if you were concerned about your child's emotions or behavior?" Doctors/mental health specialists were the least likely resource that Black mothers would pursue, when compared with the aforementioned communalistic and spiritually based resources.[47] Similar trends can be seen in Black youth who often turn to culturally relevant coping skills to deal with discrimination stress such as communalistic coping (ie, "spend time around my family"), spiritually centered coping (ie, "ask God for strength"), or emotional debriefing (ie, expressing oneself creatively by "writing poetry, songs, raps/rhymes, or short stories").[30] It can be theorized that the barriers to accessing mental health resources mentioned earlier in this article probably play some role in why BIPOC youth choose to utilize community-level resources to deal with mental health issues as opposed to seeking professional help. However, it is important to acknowledge that culture and religion can also be protective factors.[52–54]

Cultural and religious rituals such as Ramadan in Turkish communities, Lunar New Year celebrations in Chinese communities, or funerals and graduations in Latinx and Black communities have been shown to help with emotion regulation, coping with stress, enhancing community engagement, and fostering social bonds and support systems.[54] There are also studies that illustrate how cultural factors can be protective specifically against anxiety in children of color.[52,53,55] For example, Suarez and colleagues[53] found that foreign-born Latinos living in the United States had the lowest rates of childhood-onset anxiety and had a much later age of onset (usually in adulthood) of anxiety disorders compared with US-born Latino and US-born White participants. In Black cultures, reinforcing messages of cultural pride in Black families is also associated with lower anxiety in children, with a dose-dependent relationship.[52] Therefore, it is necessary for providers to understand and acknowledge both the benefits and obstacles that culture and religion pose to BIPOC youth with mental health difficulties.

### Social Media

Social media can provide groups and communities to help many youth meet developmentally appropriate needs. However, social media is also poorly monitored and can induce stress, body dissatisfaction, cognitive overload, low sense of well-being, an increased likelihood to isolate self, and feelings of anxiety and depression.[56] Race has a unique component in the experiences of social media use and adolescents of color. Social media provides community engagement to help adolescents of color strengthen their racial identity, advocate for social justice, and establish safe spaces to talk about their lived experiences.[57] However, Internet racial discrimination also poses a risk. There are 2 forms of social media racial discrimination: individual and vicarious individual social media discrimination is directed toward the person utilizing the Internet.[57] Vicarious racial discrimination is defined by observed maltreatment toward others in the same or another racial minority group on the Internet.[57] Social media racial discrimination (individual and vicarious) has been found to be significantly related to depressive symptoms, anxiety, and alcohol use disorder.[56–59] Black youth spend much more time online than non-Black adolescents for various reasons, despite increased barriers to Internet usage in the home, which leaves them much more susceptible to witnessing and internalizing these messages.[58,59]

A recent study was conducted during the COVID-19 pandemic (Fall 2020–Winter 2021) to assess the impacts of social media discrimination and racial justice involvement on adolescents of color (ie, African American, East/Southeast Asian American, Indigenous, and Latinx).[57] They found that 94% of their sample experienced vicarious social media discrimination and 79% experienced individual social media discrimination. Furthermore, they found that Black youth reported higher levels of social media racial discrimination compared with the other racial/ethnic minority groups.[57]

### Substance Use and Anxiety

Anxiety disorders have long been associated with substance use—either as a side effect or as a form of self-treatment. Substance use, specifically marijuana use, has been generally associated, by both the public and providers, with increased prevalence of anxiety disorders. Although patients diagnosed with anxiety disorders have a higher prevalence of marijuana use, no causal relationship has been established.[60] The use of marijuana and the development of anxiety disorders remains a complex area of study, specifically in BIPOC youth.

When reviewed under the lens of minoritized youth, African American boys diagnosed with social anxiety and separation anxiety disorders demonstrate a lower likelihood of utilizing substances—while those with generalized anxiety disorder and panic disorder demonstrate an increased propensity for substance use. This was also seen in adolescent White youth.[61] However, this correlation was not demonstrated in African American girls or Latinx youth.[61] These discrepancies may be related to differences in cultural and familial structures but, nonetheless, it further demonstrates the need for stratification of samples by gender and race while studying substance use and anxiety disorders in adolescents.[61,62]

### TREATMENT CONSIDERATIONS
### Psychotherapies

Treatment of anxiety disorders relies heavily on evidence-based protocols and interventions, which are often centered on cognitive behavioral therapy (CBT). These interventions focused on teaching skills to help patients identify the impact of thoughts, feelings, and behaviors as a means of reducing negative affect and in order to increase mood and a youth's ability to function. Although there is much research on the impact and effectiveness of this intervention in the general population, there is limited research on its effectiveness particularly in BIPOC youth. CBT has been shown to be effective among Black children when provided in a culturally relevant way[63]; however, studies looking specifically at racial differences in effectiveness of treatment are limited. Furthermore, most studies focusing on the efficacy of treatment do not consider race due to difficulties with sample size.[64] In a multisite child/adolescent anxiety multimodal study , it was noted that, in particular, Black youth were identified to be less engaged in therapy services and demonstrated less mastery of the CBT-based skills as reported by their therapist. It was also noted that they were less likely to receive any significant remission of their anxiety symptoms based on these protocols.[50]

Utilizing facets of dialectical behavior therapy (DBT) may serve as a method to better support BIPOC youth with adaptations focused on accepting that patients are doing their best and can make changes to improve and develop a life worth living. Unfortunately, no studies or treatment outcomes on the effects of DBT on Black populations are published.[65] Fortunately, Pierson and authors[65] posit the use of DBT with a lens of

**Table 3**
**Brief behavioral therapy in the pediatric setting**

| | Adaptations/Recommendations | |
|---|---|---|
| Evidence based therapies:<br>CBT<br>DBT | Assess for nonessential components of evidence based protocols and adjust to remove barriers to care | Increasing family involvement in sessions<br>Reducing the frequency of therapy sessions to accommodate family schedules<br>Consider telehealth appointments |
| Health system adaptations | Deploy intervention in primary care settings—less stigmatizing and more accessible | Due to the presence of somatic symptoms |
| Intervention-level adaptations | Consider the comorbidity treatment of anxiety and depression and avoid segregation of these 2 treatment protocols because this could be a barrier to families because these diagnoses often include a family history with multiple family members needing treatment of these disorders | BBT focuses on reducing youth's avoidance of the threat and increasing approach behaviors to increase rewarding life experiences.<br>Target mechanisms that cut across symptoms to increase efficiency of intervention |
| Provider-level interventions | Focus on decreasing provider burden | Increase in cultural humility, unconscious bias, training for providers on how to engage in sensitive race/ethnicity-related topics. Use youth and family metaphors |
| Patient-level interventions | | Increase parental involvement<br>Match patients to provider of preferred race/ethnicity (as preferred and available)<br>Utilize community members and group interventions to increase social support and reduce stigma |

critical race psychology (eg, analyzing psychological theories from the perspective of critical race theory) could stand to serve the Black community. Exploration of the effects of DBT on BIPOC youth may prove worthwhile. It is imperative for providers to determine what components of anxiety treatment protocols are essential to clinical improvement and which can be adapted in order to remove barriers to access of that service[50] (**Table 3** for potential adaptations and recommendations).

## PSYCHOPHARMACOLOGY

Pharmacotherapy for children with anxiety has been a point of interest for researchers the past several years as medications have advanced, specifically if there are differences between ethnic and racial groups. Few studies have reviewed the differences between racial groups.[66] Although medication effects have not been noted to differ among racial groups, it has been noted that Black youth are less likely to be prescribed medications for their anxiety disorders.[67] Additionally, Black children on Medicaid were less likely to be prescribed psychotropic medications and were less likely to meet Medicaid eligibility when compared with similar users who were White.[67,68]

Treatment of anxiety disorders finds the most benefit from a combination of CBT and pharmacologic agents. When comparing combined versus individual regimens, it is noted that Black and White youth seem to have similar remission rates; however, when Black children were rated by White providers, they were found to be less engaged and less likely to remit.[69] Similarly, Latinx populations were more likely to be rated as having increased levels of posttreatment anxiety and less likely to reach remission even when controlling for lower socioeconomic status and home living situation.[70]

---

**Box 5**
**Helpful resources for patients and families**

- National Alliance on Mental Health-NAMI-Identity and Cultural Dimensions: https://www.nami.org/Your-Journey/Identity-and-Cultural-Dimensions

- American Foundation of Suicide Prevention-Supporting Diverse Communities: Mental Health and Suicide prevention. https://afsp.org/supporting-diverse-communities

- Inclusive Therapists: inclusivetherapists.com

- AAKOMA Project: Mental Health Needs for Youth of Color https://aakomaproject.org/

- Black Mental Health Alliance-https://blackmentalhealth.com/

- Asian Mental Health Collective: https://www.asianmhc.org/

- Center for Native American Youth-https://www.aspeninstitute.org/programs/center-for-native-american-youth/

- Latinx Therapy: https://latinxtherapy.com/

- National Queer and Trans Therapist of Color Network: https://nqttcn.com/en/

- MindRight—(https://www.mindright.io/) Culturally responsive, daily coaching over text message for people who want to talk, judgment free

- Applications
  - Headspace
  - MindShift—12 y and older, Free
  - BoosterBuddy—12 y and older, Free
  - Moodtrack, US$0.99 one-time fee
  - Smiling mind, free-meditation, and mindfulness

**Box 6**
**Clinics care points**

- Increase psychiatric education/knowledge within pediatric/internal medicine/family medicine residency programs regarding cultural considerations for youth of color.

- There is a need for inclusiveness of identification of distress and somatic concerns in primary care and other medical settings that are able to use brief therapeutic interventions. Moreover, allowing for increased access to social support networks and therapeutic support will help to both normalize and increase the sense of connection to peers. Parents and primary care collaboration toward shared goals of child(ren), helps decrease self-stigma of parents and increase help-seeking due to familiarity and established trust between provider and parent.[48]

- It is imperative for clinicians to ensure that any interventions for anxiety are adopted in a way that allows for generalization as well as personalization to the individualized treatment needs of the patient and family being serviced. This is an important therapeutic skill that is a very culturally responsive intervention; however, it exists on a continuum in which a person can only mention race and impact as an isolated incident or is continuously engaged in a therapeutic process that allows for genuine openness and curiosity about a youth's experience.

- Broaching this allows for an increase in building and fostering therapeutic trust as well as promoting additional self-disclosure for the youth throughout their service delivery.

- The increase in race-based stress also calls for an awareness and increased ability by the clinician to be able to incorporate conversations regarding race and racism, understand its impact on the therapeutic work that a youth is able to engage in, and to be able to be proactive in these approaches. Proactively addressing these concerns within a therapeutic context specifically regarding race, ethnicity, and culture is also known as broaching.[73,74]

- Focusing on barriers to an individual's thriving is critically important and recommended for all clinicians. This includes identifying the presence of social determinants of mental health and assisting patients and parents with access to basic needs such as food and shelter in order to allow them the opportunity to engage in additional mental health supports.[33]

- It is also important to recognize the factors that contribute to a patient's resilience and thriving in order to be able to identify and target similar interventions for other groups of adolescents and further strengthen those individual factors.

- Normalizing conversations around mental health in schools and community settings via community interventions can increase the destigmatization of mental health and psychotherapy.

- More parental education on the risks, benefits, and perceived need for medication management for pediatric mental health issues has the potential to help combat some of the racial disparities observed in the utilization of mental health services by BIPOC youth.[51]

- An increase in the representation of racial/ethnic minorities in psychological and psychiatric workforce can also help to minimize provider-patient racial discordance and allow minoritized youth or their families to feel more comfortable seeking treatment.

- With the knowledge that communities of color rely more heavily on communalistic and spiritual-based resources such as pastors and teachers, community outreach in the form of education and training is one way that mental health professionals can bridge the gap in access, reduce racial/ethnic disparities in this line of work, and better meet the needs of our BIPOC youth more intentionally.

- The DSM-5-TR Cultural Formulation and Cultural Formulation Interview provide a framework to gather information regarding cultural identities and intersectionality.[24]

- The AACAP Practice Parameters for Cultural Competence in Child and Adolescent Psychiatric Practice provides guidelines for developing cultural humility in your work with all children and adolescents.[75] Cultural Competence Practice Parameter 1 (aacap.org)

- The American Psychological Association Multicultural Guideline: An Ecological Approach to Context, Identity, and Intersectionality,[76] https://www.apa.org/about/policy/multicultural-guidelines
- National Association of Social Work Standards and Indicators for Cultural Competence in Social Work Practice [77] https://www.socialworkers.org/LinkClick.aspx?fileticket=7dVckZAYUmk%3D&portalid=0

## CULTURAL HUMILITY IN CLINICIANS

The disparities within the treatment of mental health in minority populations have been well documented; yet these disparities are still present. Improving disparities by shaping a diverse mental health workforce with cultural humility remains our goal. The foundation for this is to ensure that there is an opportunity to better support BIPOC youth with providers of similar experiences and sociocultural perspectives, which has been illustrated to have a positive impact.[45] As of 2016, researchers continue to illustrate how the BIPOC workforce remains underrepresented in comparison to the US census with Latinx providers at 5.8% versus 17.8%, Black providers at 4.4% versus 13.3%, and American Indian/Alaska Native/Native Hawaiian/Pacific Islander providers at 0.2% versus 1.5%; emphasizing the need for increased numbers of underrepresented pediatric mental health providers in a field with already increased need.[71] These numbers did not significantly differ for practicing psychologists with Latinx providers at 5% and Black providers at 4%.[72] It is worthwhile to explore how pediatric patients work with providers that have more similarities to their patients, including cultural components because this may provide greater insight and benefit into diagnostic and treatment outcomes. See **Box 5** for more patient resources.

## FUTURE DIRECTIONS

Significant areas of research should be explored from the lens of race and gender, not only in the area of pediatric psychiatry and psychology but also within the larger medical community. There is significant literature on anxiety disorders in youth; however, it is necessary for clinicians to increase awareness and inclusivity of culture in their treatment in youth, especially youth of color. Cultural humility is a dynamic process that requires ongoing awareness, knowledge, and education. This includes increasing education of clinicians and educators across pediatric medical settings, emergency rooms, mental health clinics, in schools and in communities regarding recognition and cultural humility factors in treating youth of color. Areas that require (1) continued investigation include those of psychopharmacology and substance abuse disorders, (2) studies reviewing the impact of providers of color treating BIPOC youth to determine if significant differences can be noted from those of White providers, (3) assessing and increasing awareness of implicit bias in providers. A review of the potential impact of the intersectionality of multiple minority identities including gender and sexuality is also critical to assess the implications of development of anxiety disorders in youth.

## SUMMARY

Clinicians have an ethical responsibility to consider the impact of race-related factors on youth mental health concerns. It is imperative to do this through an intersectionality framework that allows for the many identities of the patient to be recognized, processed, and discussed to discover any impact on their anxiety symptoms. Similarly, it is critical for clinicians to understand how these identities contribute to the experience and manifestation of anxiety. Cultural humility in clinical care calls for intentionality in recognizing and reducing the disparities in mental health care for BIPOC youth with anxiety disorders. Clinicians must open the door, leave it open, and allow the youth to lead the discussion. See Clinics Points (**Box 6**), which summarizes recommendations.

## DISCLOSURE

The other authors have nothing to disclose. C.S. Al-Mateen—Springer and APA Publishing-royalties.

## REFERENCES

1. Williams Crenshaw K. Mapping the margins. Smithsonian 1997;28.
2. Morton TR, Parsons EC. #BlackGirlMagic: the identity conceptualization of Black women in undergraduate STEM education. Sci Educ 2018;102:1363–93.
3. Robertson L, Akré ER, Gonzales G. Mental health disparities at the intersections of gender identity, race, and ethnicity. LGBT Health 2021;8:526–35.
4. DuPont-Reyes MJ, Villatoro AP, Phelan JC, et al. Adolescent views of mental illness stigma: an intersectional lens. Am J Orthopsychiatry 2019;90:201–11.
5. McLean CP, Asnaani A, Litz BT, et al. Gender differences in anxiety disorders: prevalence, course of illness, comorbidity and burden of illness. J Psychiatr Res 2011;45:1027–35.
6. Chandra A, Minkovitz CS. Stigma starts early: gender differences in teen willingness to use mental health services. J Adolesc Health 2006;38:754.e1–8.
7. Lindsey MA, Joe S, Nebbitt V. Family matters: the role of mental health stigma and social support on depressive symptoms and subsequent help seeking among african american boys. J Black Psychol 2010;36:458–82.
8. Elkington KS, Hackler D, McKinnon K, et al. Perceived mental illness stigma among youth in psychiatric outpatient treatment. J Adolesc Res 2012;27: 290–317.
9. Corrigan PW, Bink AB, Schmidt A, et al. What is the impact of self-stigma? Loss of self-respect and the "why try" effect. J Ment Health 2016;25:10–5.
10. Merikangas KR, He JP, Burstein M, et al. Lifetime prevalence of mental disorders in U.S. adolescents: results from the national comorbidity survey replication-adolescent supplement (NCS-A). J Am Acad Child Adolesc Psychiatry 2010; 49:980–9.
11. Louie P, Wheaton B. Prevalence and patterning of mental disorders through adolescence in 3 cohorts of black and white Americans. Am J Epidemiol 2018; 187:2332–8.
12. Last CG, Perrin S. Anxiety disorders in african-American and white children. J Abnorm Child Psychol 1993;21(2):153–64.
13. Latzman RD, Naifeh JA, Watson D, et al. Racial differences in symptoms of anxiety and depression among three cohorts of students in the Southern United States. Psychiatry 2011;74:332–48.
14. Ginsburg GS, Silverman WK. Phobic and anxiety disorders in Hispanic and Caucasian youth. J Anxiety Disord 1996;10:517–28.
15. Enrique Varela R, Vernberg EM, Sanchez-Sosa JJ, et al. Anxiety reporting and culturally associated interpretation biases and cognitive schemas: a comparison of Mexican, Mexican American, and European American families. J Clin Child Adolesc Psychol 2004;33:237–47.

16. McLaughlin KA, Hilt LM, Nolen-Hoeksema S. Racial/ethnic differences in internalizing and externalizing symptoms in adolescents. J Abnorm Child Psychol 2007; 35:801–16.

17. Tarshis TP, Jutte DP, Huffman LC. Provider recognition of psychosocial problems in low-income Latino children. J Health Care Poor Underserved 2006;17:342–57.

18. Kenney MK ay, Thierry J. Chronic conditions, functional difficulties, and disease burden among American Indian/Alaska Native children with special health care needs, 2009-2010. Matern Child Health J 2014;18:2071–9.

19. Beidas RS, Suarez L, Simpson D, et al. Contextual factors and anxiety in minority and European American youth presenting for treatment across two urban university clinics. J Anxiety Disord 2012;26:544–54.

20. Lewis-Fernández R, Hinton DE, Laria AJ, et al. Culture and the anxiety disorders: recommendations for DSM-V. Depress Anxiety 2010;27:212–29.

21. Marques L, Robinaugh DJ, Leblanc NJ, et al. Cross-cultural variations in the prevalence and presentation of anxiety disorders. Expert Rev Neurother 2011;11: 313–22.

22. Elizur Y, Perednik R. Prevalence and description of selective mutism in immigrant and native families: a controlled study. J Am Acad Child Adolesc Psychiatry 2003;42:1451–9.

23. Stinson FS, Dawson DS, Chou SP, et al. The epidemiology of DSM-IV specific phobia in the USA: results from the national epidemiologic survey on alcohol and related conditions. Psychol Med 2007;37:1047–59.

24. American Psychiatric Association. Diagnostic and statistical manual of mental disorders, 5th edition, Text Revision. Washington, DC: American Psychiatric Association; 2022.

25. Chou T, Asnaani A, Hofmann SG. Perception of racial discrimination and psychopathology across three U.S. ethnic minority groups. Cultur Divers Ethnic Minor Psychol 2012;18:74–81.

26. Levine DS, Himle JA, Taylor RJ, et al. Panic disorder among African Americans, Caribbean blacks and non-Hispanic whites. Soc Psychiatry Psychiatr Epidemiol 2013;48:711–23.

27. Felitti VJ, Anda RF, Nordenberg D, et al. Relationship of childhood abuse and household dysfunction to many of the leading causes of death in adults: the adverse childhood experiences (ACE) study. Am J Prev Med 1998;14:245–58.

28. Thyberg CT, Lombardi BM. Examining racial differences in internalizing and externalizing diagnoses for children exposed to adverse childhood experiences. Clin Soc Work J 2022;50:286–96.

29. Zhang X, Monnat SM. Racial/ethnic differences in clusters of adverse childhood experiences and associations with adolescent mental health. SSM Popul Health 2022;17.

30. Gaylord-Harden NK, Cunningham JA. The impact of racial discrimination and coping strategies on internalizing symptoms in African American youth. J Youth Adolesc 2009;38:532–43.

31. Galán CA, Tung I, Tabachnick AR, et al. Combating the conspiracy of silence: clinician recommendations for talking about racism-related events with youth of color. J Am Acad Child Adolesc Psychiatry 2022;61:586–90.

32. Castro-Ramirez F, Al-Suwaidi M, Garcia P, et al. Racism and poverty are barriers to the treatment of youth mental health concerns. J Clin Child Adolesc Psychol 2021;50:534–46.

33. Banks A. Black adolescent experiences with COVID-19 and mental health services utilization. J Racial Ethn Health Disparities 2022;9:1097–105.

34. Centers for Disease. Control and Prevention Newsroom. New CDC data illuminate youth mental health during the COVID-19 pandemic. CDC News Press release 2022.
35. Spencer AE, Oblath R, Dayal R, et al. Changes in psychosocial functioning among urban, school-age children during the COVID-19 pandemic. Child Adolesc Psychiatry Ment Health 2021;15:1–12.
36. Singer M, Snipes C. Generations of suffering: experiences of a treatment program for substance abuse during pregnancy. J Health Care Poor Underserved 1992;3:222–34.
37. Zhou S, Banawa R, Oh H. The mental health impact of COVID-19 racial and ethnic discrimination against asian American and pacific islanders. Front Psychiatry 2021;12. https://doi.org/10.3389/fpsyt.2021.708426.
38. Ittefaq M, Abwao M, Baines A, et al. A pandemic of hate: social representations of COVID-19 in the media. Anal Soc Issues Public Policy 2022;22:225–52.
39. Penner F, Hernandez Ortiz J, Sharp C. Change in youth mental health during the COVID-19 pandemic in a majority hispanic/latinx US sample. J Am Acad Child Adolesc Psychiatry 2021;60:513–23.
40. Roche KM, Huebner DM, Lambert SF, et al. COVID-19 stressors and Latinx adolescents' mental health symptomology and school performance: a prospective study. J Youth Adolesc 2022;51:1031–47.
41. Ormiston CK, Williams F. LGBTQ youth mental health during COVID-19: unmet needs in public health and policy. Lancet 2022;399:501–3.
42. Esteves KC, Jones CW, Wade M, et al. Adverse childhood experiences: implications for offspring telomere length and psychopathology. Am J Psychiatr 2020; 177:47–57.
43. Georgiades K, Paksarian D, Rudolph KE, et al. Prevalence of mental disorder and service use by immigrant generation and race/ethnicity among U.S. Adolescents. J Am Acad Child Adolesc Psychiatry 2018;57:280–7.e2.
44. Brewer AG, Davis MM, Sheehan K, et al. Sociodemographic characteristics associated with hospitalizations for anxiety and depression among youth in Illinois. Acad Pediatr 2020;20:1133–9.
45. Yusuf HE, Copeland-Linder N, Young AS, et al. The impact of racism on the health and wellbeing of black indigenous and other youth of color (BIPOC youth). Child Adolesc Psychiatr Clin N Am 2022;31:261–75.
46. Lau M, Lin H, Flores G. Racial/ethnic disparities in health and health care among U.S. adolescents. Health Serv Res 2012;47:2031–59.
47. Murry VMB, Heflinger CA, Suiter Sv, et al. Examining perceptions about mental health care and help-seeking among rural african American families of adolescents. J Youth Adolesc 2011;40:1118–31.
48. Dempster R, Davis DW, Faye Jones V, et al. The role of stigma in parental help-seeking for perceived child behavior problems in urban, low-income african American parents. J Clin Psychol Med Settings 2015;22:265–78.
49. Senaratne R, van Ameringen M, Mancini C, et al. The burden of anxiety disorders on the family. J Nerv Ment Dis 2010;198:876–80.
50. Weersing VR, Gonzalez A, Hatch B, et al. Promoting racial/ethnic equity in psychosocial treatment outcomes for child and adolescent anxiety and depression. Psychiatric Research and Clinical Practice 2022;4:80–8.
51. Stevens J, Wang W, Fan L, et al. Parental attitudes toward children's use of antidepressants and psychotherapy. J Child Adolesc Psychopharmacol 2009;19: 289–96.

52. Bannon WM, McKay M, Chacko A, et al. Cultural pride reinforcement as a dimension of racial socialization protective of urban African American child anxiety. Fam Soc 2009;90:79–86.

53. Suárez LM, Polo AJ, Chen Chih-nan, et al. Prevalence and correlates of childhood-onset anxiety disorders among Latinos and non-latino whites in the United States. Psicol Conductual 2009;17:89–109.

54. Causadias JM, Alcalá L, Morris KS, et al. Future directions on BIPOC youth mental health: the importance of cultural rituals in the COVID-19 pandemic. J Clin Child Adolesc Psychol 2022;51:577–92.

55. Avent JR, Cashwell CS, Brown-Jeffy S. African American pastors on mental health, coping, and help seeking. Couns Values 2015;60:32–47.

56. Calancie O, Ewing L, Narducci LD, et al. Exploring how social networking sites impact youth with anxiety: a qualitative study of facebook stressors among adolescents with an anxiety disorder diagnosis. Cyberpsychology 2017;11. https://doi.org/10.5817/CP2017-4-2.

57. Tao X, Fisher CB. Exposure to social media racial discrimination and mental health among adolescents of color. J Youth Adolesc 2022;51:30–44.

58. Rideout V, Alexis L, Ellen W. Children media and raceMedia use among white,-black. Hispanic and Asian American children 2011;1–24.

59. Tynes BM, Umaña-Taylor AJ, Rose CA, et al. Online racial discrimination and the protective function of ethnic identity and self-esteem for african american adolescents. Dev Psychol 2012;48:343–55.

60. Stoner SA. Effects of marijuana on mental health: anxiety disorders. In: Alcohol & Drug. Washington: Abuse Institute, University of Washington; 2017. p. 1–6.

61. Ohannessian CM. Anxiety and substance use during adolescence. Subst Abus 2014;35:418–25.

62. Casper RC, Belanoff J, Offer D. Gender differences, but No racial group differences, in self-reported psychiatric symptoms in adolescents. J Am Acad Child Adolesc Psychiatry 1996;35:500–8.

63. Ezawa ID, Strunk DR. Differences in the delivery of cognitive behavioral therapy for depression when Therapists work with black and white patients. Cognit Ther Res 2022;46:104–13.

64. Weisz JR, Jensen-Doss A, Hawley KM. Evidence-based youth psychotherapies versus usual clinical care: a meta-analysis of direct comparisons. Am Psychol 2006;61:671–89.

65. Pierson AM, Arunagiri V, Bond DM. You didn't cause racism, and you have to solve it anyways": antiracist adaptations to dialectical behavior therapy for white Therapists. Cogn Behav Pract 2022;29:796–815.

66. Walkup JT, Albano AM, et al. Or a combination in childhood anxiety. Anxiety 2008; 359:2753–66.

67. Zito JM, Safer DJ, DosReis S, et al. Racial disparity in psychotropic medications prescribed for youths with medicaid insurance in Maryland. J Am Acad Child Adolesc Psychiatry 1998;37:179–84.

68. Zito JM, Safer DJ, Zuckerman IH, et al. Effect of Medicaid eligibility category on racial disparities in the use of psychotropic medications among youths. Psychiatr Serv 2005;56:157–63.

69. Gordon-Hollingsworth AT, Becker EM, Ginsburg GS, et al. Anxiety disorders in caucasian and african American children: a comparison of clinical characteristics, treatment process variables, and treatment outcomes. Child Psychiatry Hum Dev 2015;46:643–55.

70. Taylor JH, Lebowitz ER, Jakubovski E, et al. Monotherapy insufficient in severe anxiety? Predictors and moderators in the child/adolescent anxiety multimodal study. J Clin Child Adolesc Psychol 2018;47:266–81.
71. Wyse R, Hwang W-T, Ahmed AA, et al. Diversity by race, ethnicity, and sex within the US psychiatry physician workforce. Acad Psychiatr 2020;44:523–30.
72. Lin L, Stamm K, Christidis P. *Demographics of the U.S. Psychology workforce findings from the 2007-16*. Washington, DC: American Community Survey American Psychological Association Center for Workforce Studies; 2018.
73. Day-Vines NL, Wood SM, Grothaus T, et al. Erratum: broaching the subjects of race, ethnicity, and culture during the counseling process (Journal of Counseling & Development (2007) 85 (401-409)). J Counsel Dev 2016;94:123.
74. Day-Vines NL, Cluxton-Keller F, Agorsor C, et al. The multidimensional model of broaching behavior. J Counsel Dev 2020;98:107–18.
75. Pumariega AJ, Rothe E, Mian A, et al. Practice parameter for cultural competence in child and adolescent psychiatric practice. J Am Acad Child Adolesc Psychiatry 2013;52:1101–15.
76. American Psychological Association. Multicultural guidelines: an ecological approach to context, identity. In: and intersectionality2017. Washington, DC: American Psychological Association; 2017. p. 6–13.
77. Workers NA of S. Cultural Competence in Social Work Practice. 2015.

# Moving?

## Make sure your subscription moves with you!

To notify us of your new address, find your **Clinics Account Number** (located on your mailing label above your name), and contact customer service at:

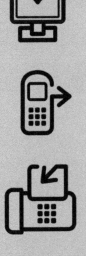

**Email: journalscustomerservice-usa@elsevier.com**

**800-654-2452** (subscribers in the U.S. & Canada)
**314-447-8871** (subscribers outside of the U.S. & Canada)

**Fax number: 314-447-8029**

**Elsevier Health Sciences Division**
**Subscription Customer Service**
**3251 Riverport Lane**
**Maryland Heights, MO 63043**

Printed and bound by CPI Group (UK) Ltd, Croydon, CR0 4YY

03/10/2024

01040466-0016